KEY TOPICS

IN **SOCIAL SCIENCES**

AN A–Z GUIDE FOR STUDENT NURSES

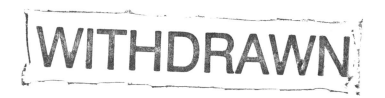

KEY TOPICS
IN SOCIAL SCIENCES

AN A–Z GUIDE FOR STUDENT NURSES

Mark Walsh

MA, BA (Hons), PGCE, RMN

Lantern

ISBN 9781908625496

Published in 2018 by Lantern Publishing Ltd

Lantern Publishing Ltd, The Old Hayloft, Vantage Business Park, Bloxham Rd, Banbury
OX16 9UX, UK

www.lanternpublishing.com

British Library Cataloguing in Publication Data

A catalogue record for this book is available from the British Library

The authors and publisher have made every attempt to ensure the content of this book is up to date and accurate. However, healthcare knowledge and information is changing all the time so the reader is advised to double-check any information in this text on drug usage, treatment procedures, the use of equipment, etc. to confirm that it complies with the latest safety recommendations, standards of practice and legislation, as well as local Trust policies and procedures. Students are advised to check with their tutor and/or mentor before carrying out any of the procedures in this textbook.

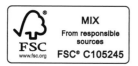

Typeset by Medlar Publishing Solutions Pvt Ltd, India
Cover design by Andrew Magee Design Ltd
Artwork by Hilary Strickland
Printed in the UK by The Complete Product Company Ltd
Distributed by NBN International, 10 Thornbury Rd, Plymouth, PL6 7PP, UK

Contents

Preface

Welcome to *Key Topics in Social Sciences*!

Developing a greater understanding of social science probably isn't the reason you chose a nurse training course and you might be wondering why you have to spend precious time trying to get to grips with social science concepts, terminology and theories. If you haven't studied social science yet, it can at first seem unfamiliar, vague and disconnected from your everyday life as a student nurse. Enthusiastic social science tutors can also forget that the words that trip off their tongues may sound obscure and meaningless to student nurses who have to cover a broad range of subjects during their degree courses. If you are new to social science, you may approach it feeling like an outsider being forced to jump through pointless hoops and fill your head with 'jargon'. In reality, studying social science is helpful and isn't as pointless or difficult as you might think at the start.

Social science concepts and theories play an important part in helping us to make sense of the complexities of everyday life, the experiences of the people you will be caring for and the world(s) and cultures they come from. As in the natural sciences, the terminology and concepts of social science do have a useful function because they enable us to think and talk about the man-made aspects of everyday life and our experiences of it. They will give you a way in to make sense of your own and other people's psychological and emotional experiences and also help you to gain a better perspective on how society more broadly can influence a person's opportunities, health choices and experiences. It might seem difficult at first, but it's important to get to grips with the 'jargon' and to learn the language of social science so that you can incorporate this into the way you think and practise as a nurse.

There are a lot of specialist social science books, dictionaries, encyclopaedias, journals and web resources out there. I suspect that your university library has a fairly good selection available. You should make use of them when you need to and have the time. The reason for this book and its A–Z format is that many student nurses don't have the time or energy to read whole social science books, carry out extensive literature reviews or hunt down obscure articles (however helpful they might be). This is a bit of a short-cut, designed to quickly get you started on new topics, to point you in the right direction in your essays and to streamline the task of building up your social science knowledge. The entries in the book don't tell you everything there is to know about a topic. They provide a way in and get you started. Treat them like a launchpad or a quick briefing that you can follow up. To make this easier, there are some 'See also' suggestions at the end of each entry. These are concepts or theories that are linked to the issue or term you have just read about. You will soon start to see the connections and have ideas about how to incorporate them into your essays. The 'Further reading' suggestions that follow provide you with a more detailed source of information on the topic if you want, and have the time, to follow this up. So, as well as saving you time, the A–Z style of the book is also trying to help you see the pathways and connections that exist between concepts, theories and terminology in the social sciences. You don't have to always follow these pathways and, hopefully, your curiosity and interest will lead you to spot and follow new pathways as you incorporate social science into your thinking and nursing practice.

Good luck with your efforts to make sense of and learn from the social sciences. It is worth it when you realise that you are able to see and understand the challenges you face and the experiences you have, in new and different ways. I am hopeful that this book will spark your enthusiasm and get you started on your exploration of the social sciences.

Mark Walsh
March 2018

About the author

Mark Walsh is a social science tutor and specialist mental health mentor who works with students taking university and further education courses. He is an experienced mental health nurse, tutor and textbook writer.

Acknowledgements

The publishers would like to thank the following former students who contributed to the development of this book by reviewing draft contents and sample material. We have listed the universities they were attending during this process, although they have graduated and registered as nurses since then.

Arefa Begum – University of Wolverhampton

Sarah Brown – University of Leeds

Harriet Davies (formerly Bradfield) – University of Cumbria

Stefan Franks – Open University

Age and ageing

Age is a flexible construct that carries different meanings, and is employed in differing ways, in the biomedical and social sciences. Social scientists treat age and ageing as social constructs. They are seen to carry culturally-based meanings about biological development and chronological age that impact on the organisation and experience of social life.

Chronological age and biological ageing

Age is often seen to be a natural, neutral fact or feature of the population. It's seen by many people as just a way of summarising how long a person, or a section of the population, has been alive. Similarly, in biological terms 'ageing' is a natural, unavoidable process. Social scientists, however, point out that the social and cultural meanings of 'age' and 'ageing' also have a considerable impact on a person's opportunities and experiences across the human lifespan.

Social and cultural aspects of age and ageing

Social scientists view 'age' and 'ageing' as social constructs rather than as naturally occurring or scientifically objective phenomena. They draw attention to 'age hierarchies' that exist in many societies. The age-based stages of childhood and youth are valued much more than old age in the age hierarchies of many western societies, for example. Arbitrary age-related divisions are also imposed to mark different stages of life ('infancy', 'childhood', 'adolescence', 'middle age', etc.), to restrict or give access to different behaviours and experiences (e.g. drinking, sex, criminal responsibility) and impact on an individual's rights, responsibilities and the expectations society imposes on them. In many developed western societies, culturally negative ideas about older people and the so-called 'ageing process' also lead to prejudice and unfair discrimination or 'ageism' that has a negative impact on the opportunities and experiences of older people. Health and social care workers need to be conscious of age-related stereotypes that can cause them to overlook the particular needs, strengths and abilities an individual has. They should always avoid making assumptions or taking decisions that are based on age-related prejudice and discrimination.

See also – Discrimination; Prejudice; Social constructionism

Further reading

Phillipson, C. (2013) *Ageing* (Key Concepts series). Cambridge: Polity.

Agency

Agency is a sociological concept that describes the ability people have to act or make decisions, either individually or collectively. More specifically, social scientists and philosophers use the concept of agency to refer to the power or ability of an individual to act freely or make decisions independently in a particular environment or situation.

There is a long-standing and ongoing debate within the social sciences about the extent to which an individual can have 'agency' within the social structures that define society and impact on their life experiences. The key issue is: to what extent are we able to act on and influence the social structures, institutions and systems (social class, gender, ethnicity) that constitute and characterise society? In relation to health and social care, this debate focuses on the extent to which individuals within society possess and can use agency to affect their life chances and health experiences, for example.

Social scientists who use a social action approach to understanding human social behaviour tend to argue that people have a significant degree of agency even if this is influenced by other factors such as their cultural background, gender, social class and ethnicity, for example. In this sense, people have the power and autonomy to make choices about their health and social behaviour and can influence the direction of their life.

By contrast, social scientists who use a structuralist approach in their analysis of human social behaviour tend to argue that structural factors such as social class, age, gender, ethnicity and sexuality (CAGES) play a more powerful role in determining an individual's life chances and experiences, and suggest that individual agency to resist or effect these social forces is limited.

See also – Age; Ethnicity; Gender; Sexuality; Social action and social structure; Social class

Further reading

Haralambos, M. and Holborn, M. (2013) *Sociology Themes and Perspectives*, 8th edition. London: Collins Education.

Alienation

Alienation is a concept that describes the separation of an individual or group of people from modern society or some aspect of their sense of self. People who are alienated are said to feel powerless and experience a sense of helplessness about their position and role in modern society.

The sociological debate about alienation began with the work of Karl Marx and Friedrich Engels (1988). They argued that workers in capitalist societies are inevitably socially and economically alienated from what they produce and why they produce it, because they are exploited. The division of labour, and the hierarchies that develop in society, mean that workers lose control of their lives and their selves because they lack control over their work. Consequently, workers are unable to become autonomous, fully realised human beings. From this perspective, working for the benefit of a capitalist elite, rather than for personal or public good, prevents an individual from becoming a social being because he or she is unable to escape economic exploitation. It is because the workers are deprived of the right to think of themselves as fully autonomous and the director of their own actions that they lose the ability to shape their own life and determine their destiny.

Marx's arguments about alienation being an inevitable consequence or condition of capitalist societies were further developed by other sociologists during the late nineteenth and early twentieth centuries. For example, Georg Simmel and Ferdinand Tönnies argued that social changes under capitalism resulted in significant shifts in the character of human relationships. Pre-modern social connections between people based on familial and community relationships were, they argued, becoming more impersonal, money orientated and transactional. As modern society became less responsive to the individuality of each member, alienation increased. By the mid-twentieth century, the American sociologist C. Wright Mills (1951) was describing how modern consumption-capitalism was alienating people further by pushing people to use their personality in superficial ways to make and maintain social relationships.

Social scientists now see alienation as incorporating a number of elements or characteristics, including:
- powerlessness – that is, a perceived gap between what a person would like to do and what they feel capable of doing
- meaninglessness – that is, not understanding what is happening or might happen in a person's life
- normlessness – that is, a lack of clarity about what the rules for social behaviour are as well as a lack of regulation or response to socially unacceptable behaviour
- weaker social relationships within families, communities and groups in society, resulting in loss of identity and social cohesion
- greater social isolation of individuals within fragmented, less supportive communities and between segregated communities and society, to the extent that much of an individual's everyday social interaction is with strangers with whom they have no ongoing social relationship.

Long-term conditions, including mental health problems, substance misuse and physical disabilities, as well as old age, poverty and social exclusion, can result in people becoming temporarily or permanently alienated from their families, communities and society generally. Nurses frequently come across people who have a sense of alienation and disconnection from others and need to take this into account when providing support and trying to engage such people in care and treatment plans.

See also – Marxism; Mental illness; Society

References and further reading

Haralambos, M. and Holborn, M. (2013) *Sociology Themes and Perspectives*, 8th edition. London: Collins Education.

Marx, K. and Engels, F. (1988) *The Economic and Philosophic Manuscripts of 1844*. Amherst, NY: Prometheus Books.

Wright Mills, C. (1951) *White Collar: the American middle classes*. New York: Oxford University Press.

Altruism

Altruism is action or behaviour that is done with the conscious intention of helping another person or group of people. In basic terms, altruism is the opposite of selfishness.

As a philosophical term, altruism was first used by the French philosopher, and pioneer of sociology, Auguste Comte. He used the term as an antonym, or opposite, of egoism. The concept of altruism is now used in biological science as well as in philosophy and social science.

Evolutionary biologists who study animal behaviour (ethology) and social evolution see altruism as a behaviour that increases the evolutionary 'fitness' of an individual whilst decreasing the fitness of the person carrying it out. This doesn't seem to make much sense in evolutionary terms. However, it's argued that altruism does make evolutionary sense for kinship selection reasons (promoting the interests of children, relatives and other 'connected' people), to promote a person's vested interests and in-group cooperation if the person believes they'll eventually benefit and to trigger 'reciprocal altruism' (the 'you scratch my back and I'll scratch yours' approach). The problem that evolutionary biologists have is explaining how altruism evolved in the first place given that a first emotionally empathetic person would have been exploited to death by the other non-empathetic individuals existing at the same time. How did altruism come to have any evolutionary use or value?

From a psychological perspective, altruism is a psychological state motivated by the desire to increase another person's welfare – that is, to help someone. In contrast to the evolutionary biology argument, the altruistic person doesn't set out, or expect, to benefit. However, many psychologists dispute the suggestion that altruism is always, or needs to be, self-sacrificial. They argue that altruistic behaviour may be motivated to benefit the self (including reducing their own discomfort or distress), to benefit members of a group to which a person belongs or supports, or to express or uphold a moral principle they believe in. In these ways, there are personal gains

from behaving altruistically. Despite this, empathy-based altruism can be motivated by the selfless desire to reduce suffering and help another. A person with empathetic concern will help another, even though they could avoid doing so. A person lacking empathetic concern will not help unless it's difficult or impossible to avoid doing so. Psychologists tend to see altruism as being expressed through prosocial behaviours (helping, comforting, sharing, cooperating, community service, etc). Voluntarily choosing to help others is connected to improved physical and mental health, higher life satisfaction and longevity. However, feeling stressed by the needs of others can also have a negative effect on a person's health and wellbeing. This is reduced if the person helping is aware of and focuses on the gratitude others show towards them. This virtuous cycle of doing good and then feeling good is sometimes referred to as 'the helper's high'.

From a sociological perspective, altruism is about behaviour or action that promotes the common good. It is concerned with ways of 'building the good society' and is also sometimes referred to as 'social sympathy'. Altruism is typically seen as community-focused action (charitable, philanthropic and prosocial activity) that contributes to the greater public good, including the social structure, organisation and processes of a society. Creating and supporting public institutions, free blood, organ and egg/sperm donation services and welfare provision are examples of group and societal level altruism. It is possible to see these kinds of activity as ways of making a selfless contribution to society and the collective social good but they are also seen by some as examples of enlightened self-interest. The benefits may not be immediate or direct but giving blood as a free 'gift', for example, is more likely to promote and maintain positive social relations and a sense of community that would be absent or diminished if people were paid to donate their blood so that it became a transaction-based activity (Titmuss, 1971). The same argument applies to egg and sperm donation, surrogacy and organ donation. Whilst these actions may be psychologically motivated, the altruistic nature of such behaviour also has an important social component and consequences.

Altruism has long been seen as a good thing, even if some evolutionary biologists and psychologists are baffled by the apparently irrational thinking that underpins it. However, recent work in this area has also highlighted the dangers of extreme or pathological altruism. This is well-intentioned behaviour that either causes more harm than good or which does the altruistic person harm. For example, people who slip into a 'compulsive helper' role may end up disempowering those they believe they are helping, contrary to their good intentions. Similarly, people in helping and caring work roles, such as nurses and other healthcare workers, may lose sight of their own needs and end up experiencing depression and burnout through their selfless but ultimately self-destructive efforts to meet the needs of others. On a broader scale, inappropriate interventions and social policies that aim to support or provide aid for disadvantaged communities can worsen rather than improve the situation if the community doesn't want the 'help' or lacks the capacity to make use of it in a positive, sustainable way.

See also – Empathy

Reference and further reading

Singer, P. (2015) *The Most Good You Can Do: how effective altruism is changing ideas about living ethically.* New Haven, CT: Yale University Press.
Titmuss, R. (1971) *The Gift Relationship: from human blood to social policy.* New York: Pantheon Books.

Anti-psychiatry

> Anti-psychiatry is a movement, and a perspective, that argues that psychiatric explanation of, and treatments for, mental distress are invalid and do more harm than good.

The anti-psychiatry movement developed in the 1960s and 70s as a protest against the theory and allegedly oppressive practices of biomedical psychiatry. People who saw themselves as belonging to this movement rejected the concept of 'mental illness' as a biological entity, arguing that psychiatric diagnoses such as 'schizophrenia' and 'manic depression' are scientifically invalid. Their counterargument is that the psychological distress and behavioural difficulties associated with 'mental illness' can instead be seen as perfectly understandable and reasonable responses to the extreme stresses of everyday life, alienation and relationship traumas that some people experience. Alongside this, some anti-psychiatry supporters also saw psychiatry as having a social control function, labelling people who were 'difficult' and 'challenging' as 'mentally ill' to discredit them and the way they questioned 'normal' or orthodox society.

Thomas Szasz (1961), a psychotherapist, and R.D. Laing (1960), a psychiatrist, are seen as prominent members of the early anti-psychiatry movement. Laing's book *The Divided Self* (1960) argues that psychotic disorders, particularly schizophrenia, are systematic and understandable ways of thinking that produce rational strategies for coping with threatening social environments. This challenges the orthodox psychiatric view that psychotic thinking is disordered, irrational and fragmented. Similarly, Szasz (1961) argued that the experiences psychiatrists label (diagnose) as 'mental illness' are, in fact, 'problems in living' that some people encounter because they don't live by expected social rules and norms. Szasz also objected strongly to the legal powers psychiatrists have to involuntarily detain and treat people in hospital, seeing this as an abuse of state power over the individual.

The anti-psychiatry approaches of Szasz and Laing are notable for the way they challenged and critiqued western psychiatry's biomedical model, its claims and previously unquestioned authority in relation to mental health. Though it was founded on a powerful critique, the anti-psychiatry movement failed to fundamentally undermine the dominance of biomedical psychiatry over the mental health field. The development and widespread use of more effective psychotropic medication, the closure of large mental asylums and the gradual acceptance and use of psychological therapies and social support as treatment methods undermined some of the criticisms levelled by the anti-psychiatry movement. Despite this, the anti-psychiatry movement has led to more critical attitudes, progressive and eclectic treatment approaches and an acknowledgement of the social impact of 'mental illness' diagnoses. Social models of mental distress and the critical psychiatry movement also draw heavily on its ground-breaking legacy of exposing and critiquing the political dimensions of psychiatry as a form of mental health practice.

See also – Alienation; Biomedical model; Mental illness; Psychiatry

References and further reading

Cromby, J., Harper, D. and Reavey, P. (2013) *Psychology, Mental Health and Distress*. Basingstoke: Palgrave Macmillan.

Laing, R.D. (1960) *The Divided Self: an existential study in sanity and madness*. Harmondsworth: Penguin Books.

Szasz, T. (1961) *The Myth of Mental Illness: foundations of a theory of personal conduct*. New York: Hoeber-Harper.

Anxiety

Anxiety refers to the feelings of unease, apprehension or fear that people experience in everyday life when they sense danger or believe something (or somebody) may be a threat to them. Anxiety is a very common, normal and understandable human response that is not usually seen as a significant problem for most people most of the time.

In addition to being associated with particular ways of thinking and feeling, anxiety also has a biological basis. It is underpinned by the biochemical changes and musculoskeletal reactions that all human beings are 'programmed' with and which result in the flight/fight/freeze responses people have when faced with sudden, acute threats. The physical symptoms of anxiety that accompany its psychological features are generally less severe but may still be unpleasant and distressing. They include headaches, nausea, trembling, fainting, tightness in the chest, tingling in the hands and feet, over-breathing and palpitations, for example.

Explaining anxiety

The nature and occurrence of anxiety can be explained in a number of ways, depending on which psychological perspective is adopted. For example, normal anxiety is seen as an 'adaptive' response to threat or danger by evolutionary and biological psychologists. They would argue that it enables people to avoid, protect or remove themselves from potentially dangerous or harmful situations. However, this doesn't explain how or why anxiety can become a problem for some people. In practice, health and social care workers need to distinguish between normal anxiety and anxiety-based behaviour that is part of an illness-based condition or disorder.

Psychologists and care workers who adopt a psychodynamic perspective tend to see anxiety as the outcome or expression of deep, unconscious psychological processes. They would argue that anxiety is an everyday experience that most people manage effectively through the use of defence mechanisms. When a person's defence mechanisms fail or become ineffective, perhaps because the person has become too stressed, for example, their anxieties leak out and are expressed in some form of psychological distress. By contrast, psychologists and care workers who adopt a cognitive behavioural therapy approach would see maladaptive learning and the reinforcement of anxiety-driven behaviour as the reason some people develop and struggle to overcome anxiety problems.

Anxiety disorders

A significant proportion of the UK population are likely to experience an anxiety disorder at some point in their life. In 2013, 8.2 million people were diagnosed with a form of anxiety disorder (Fineberg et al., 2013).

A person is said to have an anxiety disorder when their feelings of anxiety are prolonged, extreme or are too easily triggered in circumstances most people wouldn't see as anxiety-provoking. Medically defined anxiety disorders include generalised anxiety disorder, social anxiety, post-traumatic stress disorder, panic disorder and phobias.

See also – Behaviour modification; Defence mechanisms; Post-traumatic stress disorder; Psychodynamic perspective

Reference

Fineberg, N., Haddad, P., Carpenter, L., *et al.* (2013) The size, burden and cost of disorders of the brain in the UK. *Journal of Psychopharmacology*, **27(9):** 761–70.

Attachment

The concept of attachment refers to a biologically-based drive in an infant to form an enduring emotional bond with a caregiver, usually their mother, that keeps them safe and cared for while they are too young to take care of themselves. Attachment theory builds on this concept and a range of evidence about the ways attachment impacts on later development and relationships.

Attachment theories are now an important part of health and social care practice. They are particularly relevant to work with children and families in distress and people whose behavioural and mental health problems are rooted in childhood insecurities and subsequent relationship difficulties.

John Bowlby's trilogy of books entitled *Attachment and Loss* (1969, 1973 and 1980) brought the concept of attachment, and attachment theory more generally, to the attention of health and social care practitioners. He was a British psychoanalyst who saw first-hand the destructive impact of mother–child separations in post-Second World War England. Bowlby saw attachment as a feature of human evolution in which a relatively vulnerable child sought protection from his or her mother. The absence or loss of a mother or reliable caregiver had a negative impact on the child's social and emotional development. This is because, according to Bowlby, every child is motivated to achieve and maintain a sense of security – a feeling of being safe and looked after. When a child feels secure, the attachment system is deactivated and the exploratory system takes over. The availability and responsiveness of the child's mother or caregiver is critical to this process. Bowlby argued that through repeated attachment experiences, a child develops an 'internal working model' of how their interactions with their mother (or caregiver) will typically play out. This has a profound effect on their subsequent attachment behaviour.

Mary Ainsworth (2015), a colleague of John Bowlby, developed a laboratory experiment called the 'strange situation' to explore and test the concept of attachment. She was particularly interested in individual differences in the quality of mother–infant attachment. The strange situation is a twenty-minute procedure involving infants aged twelve to eighteen months and their mothers entering a room full of toys. They are observed through a one-way mirror by a psychologist who is looking at their reactions when a sequence of eight separations and reunions occur. The first separation lasts for thirty seconds. The rest last for up to three minutes. Based on how they react, the infant is classed as either securely attached or placed into one of three insecurely attached categories:

Securely attached infants show interest in the toys when the mother is in the room.

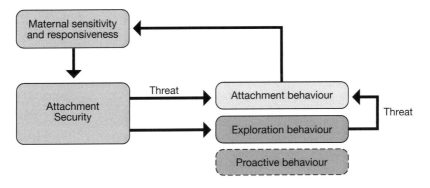

Figure 1 – An illustration of the attachment process.

Some show mild to moderate distress during separation. Importantly, the securely attached infants sought direct contact with their mother during the reunions. Any distress is quickly soothed by the mother. According to Ainsworth, this pattern of behaviour shows the child feels secure because they know their mother is available and will respond to their attachment needs.

Insecurely attached infants feel uncertain and emotionally insecure about their mother's availability and responsiveness to their attachment needs. In the strange situation they show greater interest in the toys than in their mother and are not really distressed during separations. Those who have an avoidant attachment turn away when reunited with their mothers. By contrast, infants who have a 'resistant attachment' don't really play with the toys much when their mother is present and become much more distressed when separated. They do seek out their mother on reunion but resist attempts by the mother to calm and soothe them. Ainsworth argues that these children are overly dependent and are trying to maximise their mother's attention because they are uncertain about her emotional availability and responsiveness.

Disorganised attachment is the final type of attachment relationship. Infants who have a disorganised attachment don't display a consistent strategy for dealing with attachment and separation and may seem fearful of their mother/parent. This pattern of attachment is more likely to be found in children who have experienced abuse or whose mothers have emotional difficulties themselves and do not respond to their children in an appropriate and consistent way. In these circumstances, the infant or child can't find a consistent way of dealing with their parent's erratic or frightening behaviour.

John Bowlby (1989) argued that secure attachment equips an infant with the emotional capacity to understand others and to form effective relationships at various points in their life. The capacity for attachment, based on an individual's first relationship with their parent(s) or caregivers, is seen as providing a 'blueprint' for later social and emotional development. Consequently, poor or faulty attachment may lead to deep feelings of insecurity and difficulties in forming and maintaining relationships in later life.

Attachment is an issue that interests early years and education workers, health and

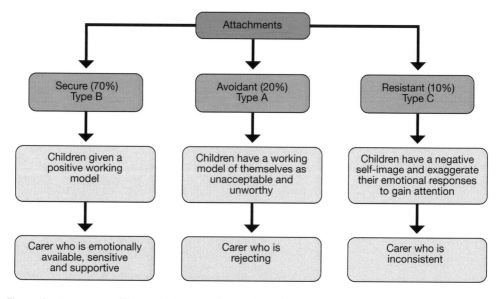

Figure 2 – A summary of Ainsworth's types of normal attachment.

social care workers supporting children and families and psychologists, counsellors and psychotherapists working with people across the lifespan. In mental health settings, attachment issues are particularly important when working with people experiencing relationship difficulties and those who have been diagnosed with a personality disorder.

See also – Autonomy; Empathy; Resilience

References

Ainsworth, M.D., Blehar, M.C., Waters, E. and Wall, S. (2015) *Patterns of Attachment: a psychological study of the strange situation*. Hove: Routledge.

Bowlby, J. (1969, 1973 and 1980) *Attachment and Loss*. New York: Basic Books.

Bowlby, J. (1989) *A Secure Base: parent–child attachment and healthy human development*. London: Routledge.

Attitudes

An attitude is a way of thinking or feeling about something. People tend to hold a variety of positive and negative attitudes about a range of issues. These express their point of view or approach to something (a person, an issue or an activity, for example) and can influence the way a person behaves.

The ABC model of attitudes best captures the link between a person's thoughts, feelings and their behaviour. It says that there are three parts to an attitude:
- Affective part – involving the person's feelings about something
- Behavioural part – the impact the attitude has on the way a person acts
- Cognitive part – the person's knowledge or belief about something.

There is a common assumption that a person's behaviour will be consistent with their attitudes. However, this doesn't always hold true – a person may express positive attitudes publicly and behave in a negative way privately, for example. Alternatively, a person may say they don't like or are frightened of a particular group of people but treat individuals from this group politely and positively in practice. Attitude strength is a better predictor of a person's likely behaviour. The stronger a person's attitude is towards something, the more likely they are to behave or act in accordance with their attitude. This is particularly the case where a person's attitudes are based on direct experience.

Attitude change

A person's attitudes are strongly influenced by their upbringing and socialisation but are never fixed or completely stable. We are constantly developing, reviewing and reshaping our attitudes in response to the interactions, communication and experiences we have with others in society. A broad range of social influences (the media, peers, co-workers, partners, family members, etc.), as well as the individual's own motivation to achieve cognitive consistency, can lead a person to change or adjust their attitude.

Psychologists suggest that the following three psychological processes can all result in attitude change:
- Compliance – that is, people may change their attitude to comply with what they see as the expected way of behaving in a particular situation (Asch, 1956).
- Identification – that is, people may change their attitude in order to be more like someone they admire or like (a person they identify with).
- Internalisation – that is, a person's attitudes may change if they find that a new or different attitude or behaviour is more consistent with their internal and deeply-held values.

Festinger (1957) extended the study and understanding of attitude change by introducing the concept of 'cognitive dissonance' into psychology. This is the sense of unease or guilt people experience when they hold conflicting cognitions (thoughts/beliefs) or when there is an inconsistency between their attitude and their behaviour. Festinger argued that a person in this situation may be motivated to change their attitudes and beliefs in order to reduce the cognitive dissonance they are experiencing.

See also – Attitudes; Cognitive dissonance; Cognitive perspective

References

Asch, S. E. (1956) Studies of independence and conformity: a minority of one against a unanimous majority. *Psychological Monographs*, 70 (whole no. 416).
Festinger, L. (1957) *A Theory of Cognitive Dissonance*. Stanford, CA: Stanford University Press.

Attribution theory

Attribution theory focuses on how individuals explain the causes of behaviour and events.

People experience a wide range of behaviour in everyday life and are faced with the daily challenge of understanding the complex social world in which they live. Heider (1958), a German Gestalt psychologist, noted that people make sense of events by seeing or proposing 'cause and effect' relationships. Heider (1958) argued that a person might do this through:

Internal attribution

This involves attributing the cause of a person's behaviour to an enduring internal characteristic rather than to an external influence. Typically, this will involve explaining a person's behaviour in terms of their personality, character, motives or beliefs.

External attribution

This involves attributing the cause of a person's behaviour to an external situation, factor or event that is outside of the person's control and which is not located within them as a person. People often make external attributions when explaining their own behaviour.

Building on Heider's (1958) ideas and themes, Jones and Davis (1965) argued that people tend to focus on intentional behaviour when making attributions, rather than on accidental or inadvertent responses. Their so-called correspondent inference theory suggested that when a person makes an internal attribution they make links between an individual's motives and their behaviour. In effect, if we see a person behaving in a friendly way we infer they have corresponding friendly motives and are a friendly person. This is also known as dispositional attribution.

Kelley (1967) extended attribution theory further with his covariation model. This provides a method for working out whether a particular behaviour or action should be explained through an internal or external attribution. Kelley (1967) argued that we use a range of different sources of information (consensus, distinctiveness and consistency information) to determine whether a person's behaviour is internally or externally driven. Using our own observations, experience and knowledge we look for correlations between these sources of information to determine the likely cause of the person's behaviour.

Attribution theory has been used to give healthcare practitioners insights into how people explain the causes of their illness and the health outcomes of their behaviour. Finding out how a person understands the cause of their illness is therefore important in planning treatment as it impacts on treatment compliance. However, attribution theory has also been criticised as mechanistic and reductionist for assuming that people are rational, logical and systematic thinkers. It also neglects the social, cultural and historical factors that can inform and shape an individual's attributions.

See also – Memory; Motivation; Personality

References and further reading

Heider, F. (1958) *The Psychology of Interpersonal Relations.* New York: Wiley.
Hogg, M. and Vaughan, G. (2013) *Social Psychology*, 7th edition. Harlow: Pearson.
Jones, E. E. and Davis, K. E. (1965) 'From acts to dispositions: the attribution process in social psychology', in L. Berkowitz (ed.), *Advances in Experimental Social Psychology* (volume 2, pp. 219–266). New York: Academic Press.
Kelley, H. H. (1967) 'Attribution theory in social psychology'. In D. Levine (ed.), *Nebraska Symposium on Motivation* (volume 15, pp. 192–238). Lincoln, NE: University of Nebraska Press.

Authority

The concept of authority refers to the legitimate power that one person or group holds over another person or group.

A person is in a position of authority when they are able to issue commands that they have a reasonable expectation will be carried out. This will only happen if the people receiving the command believe and accept that the person issuing them is doing so legitimately. Max Weber (1925), one of the founding theorists of sociology, saw power and authority as key features of social relations at all levels of society. For example, authority is a feature of parent–child, teacher–pupil and employer–employee relations as well as in the relationships we have with healthcare professionals, law enforcement agencies and national governments. Weber identified three types of authority:

- Traditional – where power is legitimised through respect for and deference towards others because of their status. The legitimacy of traditional authority is captured in the phrase 'this is the way it has always been done'. Traditional authority is based on an allegiance to rulers not rules.
- Charismatic – where power is legitimised through devotion to a charismatic leader's special qualities. These special qualities must be supported, at least occasionally, by evidence that the person is exceptional and deserving of allegiance. If this does not happen, the charismatic leader's authority may be challenged, making this an unstable form of authority.
- Rational-legal – where power is legitimised through laws and regulations passed by democratic authorities rather than through tradition or the preferences of a charismatic individual.

Weber argued that these types of authority can exist at the same time in a society and that any one of them could become dominant.

See also – Obedience; Power

Reference and further reading

Haralambos, M. and Holborn, M. (2013) *Sociology Themes and Perspectives*, 8th edition. London: Collins Education.

Weber, M. (1925) *Economy and Society: an outline of interpretive sociology*. Berkeley, CA: University of California Press.

Autonomy

> Autonomy is a philosophical idea or concept that refers to the right to be self-governing. That is, a person who has 'autonomy' is free and capable of making decisions for themselves.

In health and social care settings, all service users are assumed to be autonomous (to have autonomy) unless they lack the mental capacity to understand and make decisions for themselves. People who have dementia, some people with mental health problems and some people with learning disabilities or a neurological (brain-based) condition, may not have the mental capacity to be autonomous.

Respect for the autonomy of each individual service user provides the foundation for the key principle of 'informed consent'. That is, care, treatment or any medical, psychological or social intervention can only proceed if the person understands what is being proposed and agrees to this. Because they have autonomy, the person has the right to decline or refuse treatment, care or intervention – even in situations where qualified and experienced practitioners recommend or advise them to accept it.

Acknowledging and respecting the individual's right to autonomy should also have a major effect on the way health and social care practitioners form relationships and interact with service users. Accepting an individual as an autonomous person means that they are an equal and that any care or therapeutic relationship with them is a partnership. It isn't acceptable for a health or social care worker to use their professional expertise and position to disempower or impose decisions on an autonomous person. There are some exceptions to this – such as where the individual lacks mental capacity – but it is generally good professional practice to ensure everything is done to respect an individual's autonomy.

See also – Agency; Attachment; Empathy; Resilience

Further reading

Barnard, A. (2017) *Developing Professional Practice in Health and Social Care*. Abingdon: Routledge.

Cuthbert, S. and Quallington, J. (2017) *Values and Ethics for Care Practice*. Banbury: Lantern Publishing.

Behaviour

Psychologists view behaviour as the observable responses a person makes, or the actions they take, in relation to specific stimuli.

In addition to investigating how learning can occur through stimulus-response associations (behavioural psychology), psychologists have also investigated and sought to explain the biological basis of human behaviour (biological psychology), the social influences on behaviour development (social learning theory) and the links between mental processes and behaviour (cognitive psychology). The development and expression of human behaviour remain a key focus of many contemporary psychologists who wish to understand connections between the human mind and how people respond and act in different situations.

Sociologists tend to focus more on patterns of behaviour within groups, communities or subcultures in a society (e.g. their routines, habits, social practices), on the way behaviours carry and convey social and cultural meanings (e.g. holding hands, greetings, behaviours in groups) and on the way that behaviour is used for social purposes such as social control, social support and social influence.

See also – Altruism; Behaviour modification; Behaviourism; Challenging behaviour

Further reading

Gross, R. (2015) *Psychology: the science of mind and behaviour*, 7th edition. London: Hodder Education.

Behaviour modification

Behaviour modification is a behavioural psychology approach to changing human behaviour using rewards to reinforce new, desirable behaviours and/or extinguish unwanted or undesirable behaviour(s). It is based on operant conditioning principles.

Psychologists and care workers can use a variety of behavioural techniques to change unwanted, maladaptive and challenging behaviours and to stimulate and shape new forms of behaviour. Often the people who are given behavioural treatments use coping strategies that are damaging to themselves or others to deal with particular situations or stresses in life. Heavy drinking or drug-taking in response to stress, or avoidance of travelling by aeroplane for fear of dying are examples of maladaptive behaviours.

The behavioural concepts of association and reinforcement can be used to trace back the origins of these kinds of behavioural and emotional problems and can help care practitioners understand an individual's behaviour.

Behaviour modification strategies

Aversion therapy is a form of classical conditioning that uses negative reinforcement to change maladaptive behaviour. Negative reinforcement involves the removal of a discouraging or negative stimulus associated with a behaviour. It has been used as a treatment for alcoholism, for example, where the person is given a drug (Antabuse) that is perfectly safe and which has no side-effects – until the person drinks alcohol. When alcohol is consumed, the person feels very unwell and may be violently sick. Over time the person learns to associate these unpleasant feelings and experiences with alcohol and stops drinking to avoid them. The same technique is used when a child's nails are painted with an unpleasant-tasting solution to deter them from biting them.

Systematic desensitisation is a technique that is often used to treat phobias. This involves reducing and ultimately removing the power of a maladaptive association by gradually exposing the person to the thing they are frightened of (Wolpe, 1958). To do this the care practitioner and the phobic person first create a 'hierarchy of fear'. The treatment stage involves gradually exposing the person to varying degrees of fear whilst also helping them to relax and cope with each exposure. The goal is for the person to face the situation or object that they are fearful of or phobic about, without worrying. Systematic desensitisation has been used effectively to help people overcome all kinds of phobias, from agoraphobia (fear of open spaces) to fear of spiders, that cause distress and disrupt people's lives.

Token economy systems are a behaviour modification strategy that use the principles of operant conditioning to stimulate or shape behaviours. Token economy systems use reinforcement (and to a lesser extent punishment) to change and shape an individual's behaviour. Typically, this involves establishing a system of 'token' rewards to reinforce desired behaviours. For example, parents and childcare workers sometimes use 'reward' stickers to encourage young children to learn to use the potty and the toilet instead of a nappy. A token economy approach has been shown to be an effective way of controlling night-time bed-wetting in children capable of bladder control (Glazener and Evans, 2002).

Token economy systems were a common feature of mental health and learning disability services until the 1980s. They were generally used to motivate and reinforce the development of self-care skills (getting dressed, having a wash, taking part in activities) in unmotivated people who had lived in large institutions such as mental hospitals for many years. Unfortunately, the 'token' would often be a cigarette or an actual token that people used to buy tobacco or cigarettes. In modern care settings, care practitioners are more likely to use social reinforcement in the form of verbal praise ('Well done, that's really great') to encourage desirable health behaviour and to build up the self-esteem and self-confidence of people who use the service.

Behaviour modification techniques are now widely used in early years and educational settings to shape and respond to children's behaviour. Many childcare workers and teachers use 'reward' charts and positive forms of speech that socially reinforce desired behaviour or effort ('Well done', 'That's really good', 'Excellent work') in the classroom or care setting. You have probably experienced this approach in your own school or college career or through the approach your parents took to bringing you up.

See also – Behaviour; Behaviourism; Operant conditioning

References and further reading

Glazener, C.M. and Evans, J.H. (2002) Simple behavioural and physical interventions for nocturnal enuresis in children. *Cochrane Database of Systematic Reviews*, 2: CD003637.

Gross, R. (2015) *Psychology: the science of mind and behaviour*, 7th edition. London: Hodder Education.

Wolpe, J. (1958) *Psychotherapy by Reciprocal Inhibition*. Stanford, CA: Stanford University Press.

Behaviourism

Behaviourism is a major psychological perspective that focuses on human behaviour and learning processes. Behaviourism was the dominant perspective in psychology during the first half of the twentieth century. It continues to be widely used in health and social care settings, but is now less influential within mainstream psychology than it once was.

The behaviourist approach in psychology focuses on behaviour that can be observed. It is sometimes also known as 'learning theory' because its basic focus is on the way that human beings learn and the impact this has on their behaviour and relationships. For example, behaviourists believe that people have to learn how to make and maintain relationships and that the way we cope with stress and pressure is also the result of what we have learnt from others. Behaviourists claim that human behaviour is:

- learnt from experience
- more likely to be repeated if reinforcement occurs.

Reinforcement is the process by which a response is strengthened and thereby reinforced.

Ivan Pavlov (1849–1936), a Russian physiologist, and B. F. Skinner (1904–90), an American psychologist, are the theorists most closely associated with the behaviourist perspective. Pavlov inadvertently discovered the principles of classical conditioning whilst he was investigating digestion processes in dogs.

B. F. Skinner made a more deliberate attempt to investigate animal learning using rats and pigeons to test his theory of instrumental learning. The learning process that he identified and demonstrated is now known as operant conditioning.

The strengths and weaknesses or limitations of the behaviourist approach to psychology are summarised in *Table 1*.

Table 1 – Strengths and weaknesses of the behaviourist approach to psychology

Strengths	Weaknesses/limitations
The behaviourist approach has been widely used to successfully modify (e.g. phobias) and motivate (e.g. weight loss) behaviour change.	Behaviourism reduces human behaviour to a simple stimulus-response level. This fails to take into account inner mental processes or wider cultural and environmental influences on behaviour.
Behavioural assessment and treatment is relatively quick, inexpensive and solution-focused.	Some care workers and psychologists are critical of behaviourism for being manipulative and for not addressing the underlying causes of an individual's problems.
Changes in behaviour can be easily measured, monitored and observed.	Behavioural treatments work well in controlled environments, especially with animals. They have a more limited application to the real-world behaviour of human beings.

See also – Behaviour modification; Classical conditioning; Operant conditioning; Reinforcement

Further reading

Fairholm, I. (2012) *Issues, Debates and Approaches in Psychology*. Basingstoke: Palgrave Macmillan.
Gross, R. (2015) *Psychology: the science of mind and behaviour*, 7th edition. London: Hodder Education.

Biomedical model

The biomedical model of health defines disease objectively by seeking and identifying physical signs that result from anatomical abnormalities and biochemical dysfunction in the body. Consequently, the biomedical model assumes that health is the 'normal' state of the human body.

The biomedical model has become the dominant approach to health in contemporary western societies and is the one that most doctors use. Because the biomedical model is now so dominant it can be difficult to believe that it is a relatively recent way of thinking about and practising 'health' care, and that a range of credible alternatives also exist.

The biomedical model of health developed alongside and makes use of scientific methods to diagnose and treat health problems. The scientific basis of biomedicine is presented as neutral, value-free and evidence-based. As such, the biomedical model used in medical practice assumes that:

- health is the absence of biological abnormality in the body
- doctors can use special 'scientific' methods and knowledge to observe the body, and to identify whether or not there are signs of any biological abnormality
- the causes of ill health are located in the individual's malfunctioning biological system
- health can be restored by using surgery and drugs to correct the malfunctions that occur.

Medical professionals trained in the theory and practices of biomedicine are considered to be the only legitimate experts in the diagnosis and treatment of disease. Alternative non-scientific practitioners and self-taught healers are also seen as lacking appropriate knowledge and expert understanding, to the extent that their practice is often considered less credible and illegitimate by those committed to biomedicine.

Acceptance of the biomedical model and its assumptions about health has resulted in particular types of healthcare services and health policies being developed in modern societies such as the UK. The structure of the National Health Service is based primarily upon the activities of specialist doctors, seeking to cure the diseases that they have identified, for example. Hospitals and other clinical, medical settings are seen as the most appropriate environments for treating serious health problems. However, there is considerable doubt that this model actually reflects reality and, increasingly, the biomedical model used by the medical profession is being challenged.

Criticisms of the biomedical model

Sociological thinking has played a significant part in the questioning of medical knowledge. In some respects, the sociology of health and illness is a sceptical response to, and critique of, what is commonly known as the biomedical model of health and illness. Social and political critiques of biomedicine and the medical profession have challenged the nature, uses and effects of medical knowledge and power in contemporary society. Criticisms have focused on:

- *The nature of biomedical knowledge* – particularly the biomedical claim that 'disease' and 'normal' functioning are naturally occurring phenomena. Sociologists argue that biomedicine should, instead, be understood as a belief system that provides a socially, historically and culturally contingent way of making sense of 'health' and 'illness' experience. What biomedicine sees as 'disease' may change over time (e.g. masturbatory insanity, homosexuality, hysteria) or may not be recognised in different cultures. Despite the implicit claims of biomedicine, 'diseases' and 'normal' functioning are not always stable, biologically-based realities.

- *The effectiveness of biomedicine* – one of the main themes in the conventional history of modern medicine is that it has developed into a highly effective way of dealing with health problems and has improved the quality of life and the longevity of the population in modern society. Sociological critics of biomedicine dispute this, arguing that the effectiveness of biomedicine has been overplayed. For example, McKeown (1976) is often quoted by sociological critics to demonstrate how the decline in mortality from infectious diseases since the nineteenth century has resulted more from social changes and public health initiatives than from developments in medical knowledge or practice.

  Ivan Illich (1976), a prominent American critic of the biomedical model, has also questioned the effectiveness of medicine, claiming that medical practices cause harm. He refers to the harmful effects of medicine as their iatrogenic consequences. Illich (1976) is critical of medical practices for contributing to illness and damage to patients' health through, for example, the development and spread of methicillin-resistant *Staphylococcus aureus* (MRSA) infection in medical settings such as hospitals. Illich (1976) also argues that medicine has indirectly had a negative impact on health by deskilling people. That is, the 'expertise' of doctors and their close control of medical knowledge and treatment skills have undermined our general ability to manage our own health and wellbeing. We are now dependent on medical 'experts' to do so.

- *The social control function of biomedicine* – sociological critics have criticised biomedicine for taking on a significant 'social control' role in contemporary society. The application of medical knowledge to 'mental illness' is seen as a good example of the way that medical practitioners have used their privileged access to highly valued 'medical knowledge' for sociopolitical purposes. Critics, including mental health service users and 'survivors', argue that 'mental illness' diagnoses that are applied by medical practitioners have more of a social control purpose than any kind of 'health' function or 'scientific' validity. In this sense, biomedical definitions of 'disease' and other ill health 'realities' are allegedly based as much on moral criteria and ethical judgements about 'normality' as on 'scientific' facts.

Arguably, the recent questioning of medical knowledge and the effectiveness of medical practices have led to a reduction of faith and trust in biomedicine and the medical profession in western societies. One consequence has been an increasing demand for non-medical, alternative or complementary forms of healthcare and greater patient control over health and care processes.

See also – Anti-psychiatry; Psychiatry; Social model of health

References and further reading

Cromby, J., Harper, D. and Reavey, P. (2013) *Psychology, Mental Health and Distress*. Basingstoke: Palgrave Macmillan.

Illich, I. (1976) *Limits to Medicine: medical nemesis – the expropriation of health*. London: Marion Boyars.

McKeown, T. (1976) *The Role of Medicine: dream, mirage or nemesis?* London: London Provincial Hospitals Trust.

(The) Body

Biologically, the human body is a physical or material structure consisting of organs, systems and processes that make possible and sustain human life. However, social scientists also recognise the body as a social and cultural entity as well as a biological one.

The body has long been seen as a distinct structure separate from the human mind and spirit, and from society more broadly. This perception of the body as detached from its environmental, cultural and social context is challenged by social scientists who see it as having an important and integral role in the human social and psychological world. For example, social scientists argue that a person's physical form and appearance is both marked by and influential at a social level. An individual's appearance – their size, shape and colour, for example – has social significance. Being black, white, female, male, physically or visually impaired, thin or large are not simply physical facts. Sociologists now argue and seek to show that our understanding of the human body is given 'meaning', or only makes sense, in the context of our awareness and application of discourses of social class, gender, age, 'race' and disability, for example. These characteristics and features of the body matter and have meaning for other people in the way they perceive and relate to the person. They also matter and impact on the person in terms of their self-image, self-esteem and their status and position in the world.

Social scientists argue that the characteristics and meanings of the human body are, unlike the narrow claims of anatomists, biological scientists and some medical professionals, also not fixed. The late twentieth and early twenty-first centuries have witnessed a huge growth in 'body project' industries that encourage people to use dieting, exercise, cosmetic surgery and body adornments such as tattooing and piercing to change, enhance and reshape the physical body, for example. Remaking the body, discovering a 'new you' and finding ways of re-presenting your body promise personal and emotional renewal as well as access to new opportunities as others see, react and respond to us differently. As a result, the human body can be sociologically analysed as a site of social meaning, or what Featherstone *et al.* (1991) call 'the visible carrier of the self'. Slowing, reversing or even stopping the ageing process is also an aspect of this area of social activity.

Postmodern philosophers such as Michel Foucault (2003) have contributed to social and cultural debates about the meaning and significance of the body by identifying it as a site for surveillance, discipline and control. Many feminist sociologists, including Simone de Beauvoir, have also identified the particular ways in which women are (de)valued, judged and controlled through society's (and their own) perceptions and responses to the female body. Within the health and social care field, the body as a social construct is debated and discussed in relation to body image, eating disorders, dieting and optimum weight and appearance, and the medical ethics of activities such as assisted suicide, surrogacy, cloning and abortion, for example.

See also – Postmodernism; Realism; Social constructionism

References

Featherstone, M., Hepworth, M. and Turner, B.S. (eds) (1991) *The Body: social processes and cultural theory*. London: SAGE Publications.
Foucault, M. (2003) *The Birth of the Clinic*, 3rd edition. Oxford: Routledge Classics.

Capitalism

Capitalism is an economic system that is based on market exchange (buying and selling goods and services) and the generation of profit for reinvestment and business growth.

Analyses of capitalism as an economic system have been a significant feature of social science theorising and debate since the nineteenth century. Karl Marx argued that capitalism was exploitive, oppressing workers and generating social inequalities that only benefited and rewarded a privileged minority – the owners of the means of production. Marx argued that whilst capitalists and workers were mutually dependent, the exploitation of the proletariat or working class by the ruling capitalist bourgeoisie would inevitably lead to class conflict. Marx argued that capitalism was doomed to fail and was, in fact, the final stage of social development before communism. He believed that a communist social and economic system would emerge to end inequalities in society. The Marxist position is a moral one in the sense that it sees the exploitation and inequalities of capitalist societies as fundamentally wrong and of greater significance than any economic benefits they may offer.

Max Weber also saw capitalism as playing a key role in shaping the structure and organisational aspects of modern society. He was particularly interested in the way capitalism was linked to the rationalisation and bureaucratisation of social life. Weber didn't believe that capitalism was either a product of, or a stage on the way to, revolutionary social change. He saw the development of capitalism as offering benefits to working class people as it encouraged and rewarded competition, innovation and experimentation with new ideas. The Weberian position is more positive and accepting of capitalism on the grounds that it provides scope for more personal freedom, democracy and economic productivity than any alternative system.

Most countries in the contemporary world have capitalist economies. Karl Marx's predictions of revolution have not come to fruition. In fact, where there have been revolutions – Russia in 1917 and China in 1949 – they have not involved a coordinated, class-conscious working class. Additionally, the collapse of Soviet and east European communism marked the end of an era of competition between the two economic systems. The growing influence and impact of globalisation and international corporate business also seems to have prevented socialism and communism from developing in the way Marx predicted. Opposition to capitalism now comes from anti-globalisation, pro-environmental and anti-capitalist movements of young, marginalised and disenfranchised groups. A core theme of these movements is that capitalism is not, and cannot become, sustainable in a world where there are finite resources, global warming and a historical pattern of veering towards economic crisis.

See also – Globalisation; Market; Marxism

Further reading

Haralambos, M. and Holborn, M. (2013) *Sociology Themes and Perspectives*, 8th edition. London: Collins Education.
Marx, K. and Engels, F. (1848/2005) *The Communist Manifesto*. London: Longman.

Causality

This concept refers to the relationship between cause and effect or the principle that one or more factors are linked to, or bring about, something else.

In everyday life, as well as in academic and clinical settings, people are constantly trying to make sense of what is going on and explain why. In essence, we are always searching for causes, looking for the reasons things happen. We want to know what might be causing a person's ill health, the reason for their mental distress or the tumour that has been revealed by a specialist scan. It's important to investigate causality because we want to be able to prevent bad things happening and to increase the chances of good things happening. That's why most people who know about the link between smoking tobacco and lung cancer don't do it. Their understanding of cause and effect – of causality – enables them to minimise their risk of experiencing lung cancer.

Causality is a central issue in both social science (theory and research) and in healthcare practice. Finding out how one factor affects another is central to developing theories, arguments and evidence as well as in diagnosing and treating people for illness and disease. Despite this, causality is rarely a simple thing to work out. Many apparently causal relationships turn out to be correlations or on closer inspection don't take into account additional, intervening variables that may also be playing a part in causing a particular outcome. This is particularly important in social science as people and everyday social situations are unpredictable and possess a level of complexity not present in carefully controlled laboratory experiments. Despite this, social scientists use the concept of causality very explicitly when they develop and test hypotheses in their research investigations and less obviously when they carry out interviews, surveys and other studies that are seeking to develop understanding of a set of circumstances, a situation or experience.

See also – Hypothesis; Research methods

Further reading

Ellis, P. (2016) *Understanding Research for Nursing Students*, 3rd edition. London: Learning Matters.

Lindsay, B. (2007) *Understanding Research and Evidence-Based Practice*. Exeter: Reflect Press.

Challenging behaviour

Challenging behaviour is any form of behaviour that is out of keeping with the expected standards or patterns of behaviour in a culture or society. In effect, it 'challenges' normal expectations and standards.

It may be the intensity, frequency or duration of the behaviour that is unusual and which puts the person or other people at risk that makes a person's behaviour 'challenging'. Challenging behaviour is usually associated with adults who have learning disabilities, mental health problems or dementia and with children experiencing 'tantrums'. Self-harm, violence, inappropriate sexual behaviour, selective incontinence, mutism and vandalism are all common types of challenging behaviour.

Behavioural analysis and treatment of challenging behaviour typically tries to identify the causes, triggers and consequences of the behaviour. Operant conditioning principles are then used to help the person develop new, more socially acceptable ways of behaving. Where a person's challenging behaviour is more self-destructive or self-defeating (drug or alcohol misuse, for example) and they are capable of developing insight into it, psychodynamic therapy may be used to expose, explore and deal with unconscious motives and influences underpinning the pattern of behaviour.

See also – Behaviour modification; Behaviourism; Operant conditioning; Psychodynamic perspective

Further reading

Emerson, E. (2011) *Challenging Behaviour*, 3rd edition. Cambridge: Cambridge University Press.

Child abuse

Child abuse occurs when a child is subjected to physical, emotional or psychological harm, sexual molestation or neglect.

Childhood abuse could involve:

- physical abuse, where injuries are deliberately inflicted or a health problem is caused by neglect
- emotional abuse, such as persistent criticism, manipulation or devaluing of the child, making unrealistic demands on or having impossibly high expectations of a child
- sexual abuse, where children view or are made to watch sexual acts, are exposed to pornography, are molested (touched sexually) or are encouraged or forced to take part in sexual acts (including intercourse and oral sex).

Detection of childhood abuse is difficult even though the impact on the child is often severe and long-lasting. It often requires inter-agency collaboration between health and social care practitioners, education staff and the police, for example. In addition, the willingness of the child, a non-abusing parent or somebody else close to the child is often needed to alert child protection professionals or school staff to suspected or actual abuse or neglect.

See also – Child development; Early experiences

Further reading

Powell, C. (2011) *Safeguarding and Child Protection for Nurses, Midwives and Health Visitors: a practical guide.* Maidenhead: Open University Press.

Child development

Child development is a very broad concept that refers to the interacting processes of physical, intellectual, emotional and social change and adaptation that occur as a person grows and develops from a dependent child into a more capable and relatively independent adolescent.

There are a number of theories of child development. Some focus on a specific aspect of child development, such as cognitive change (e.g. Piaget) or psychosexual development (Erikson), whilst others offer a more general psychological approach (e.g. Freud). Key issues in current debates about child development include:

- nature vs. nurture influences – to what extent do biological (nature) and environmental (nurture) factors influence child development and how do they interact?
- critical vs. sensitive periods – does a critical period exist in which development must occur (or be lost) or does a sensitive period exist where it is preferable, but not vital, to develop in certain ways (e.g. acquire language)?
- continuous vs. discontinuous development – do developmental changes occur in defined stages or is development more of a gradual, continuous process?

Infant development

In stage theories of child development, infancy is the first life stage following birth. It is generally thought to cover the first two years of life and is a very active stage of growth and development. Major changes occur in the physical, intellectual, emotional and social areas of a child's development during infancy.

Physical growth and development during infancy

Physical growth and development is rapid during the first infant phase of the life span. Between birth and 18 months of age a child will grow to be three times its birth weight. Rapid growth occurs in all the major body systems so that by the age of 18 months the child is very different in terms of appearance and physical capabilities to when they were born.

Some of the key physical changes that affect both the physical appearance and capability of a child in the first 18 months of life are those that occur in bone and muscles. A newborn baby has very soft bones with a high water content. Ossification, or hardening, of the bones is a gradual process that occurs sufficiently quickly in the first 18 months of life to change a baby from a floppy, helpless state to one where it can move and sit up independently. Two terms are used to describe the overall pattern in which human physical growth occurs. These are cephalocaudal (from the head downwards) and proximodistal (from the trunk outwards).

The first 18 months of life involve a spurt in the developing complexity of organs, such as the brain, and the nervous system, as well as the changes in body size and shape that can clearly be seen. By the time that the child has reached 18 months of age the physical changes that have happened will provide a basis on which motor (movement) skills can develop.

Motor development refers to the movement skills and abilities that human beings develop. Early motor development includes the emergence of:

- locomotor patterns – pulling, crawling, walking (holding on)
- non-locomotor patterns – holding head up, pushing, bending body
- manipulative skills – reaching, grasping, stacking blocks.

The movement skills that first develop during infancy are the gross motor skills. These are the basic, unsophisticated but important abilities that allow the child to control movement of their limbs, trunk and head. They give the infant the ability to reach out, hold their head up independently and roll over without help, for example. These skills are gradually added to during infancy, adolescence and adulthood as the individual develops fine motor skills. These are the sophisticated, highly skilled and controlled minor movements that many everyday activities (eating with cutlery and getting dressed, for example) depend on.

The expected pattern of physical growth during infancy is sometimes referred to as 'normal development'. Whilst children grow, i.e. put on weight and get taller, at different rates during infancy, large-scale, long-term studies of patterns of growth have provided care practitioners with data on average and normal rates of growth. This data has been used to produce centile charts of height and weight for both male and female infants.

Emotional development during infancy

An infant's early emotional development plays an important part in their future relationships with others. Ideally, an infant should have opportunities to develop feelings of trust and security during the early years of life. The process through which these feelings develop is known as attachment. This involves an infant developing a strong emotional link with their parents or main caregivers. The parent or carer response to this emotional linking is known as bonding. It is through attachment and bonding that an infant's first emotional relationship is formed.

An infant's response to others changes as they develop socially and emotionally: up to six months, the baby can be held by anyone. The baby may protest when put down by whoever is holding them. This is known as indiscriminate attachment.

Between seven and twelve months the baby is usually bonded to their parents and shows fear of strangers. This can be intense for three or four months. This is known as specific attachment.

From twelve months onwards the baby's attachments broaden to include other close relatives and people whom they see frequently. This is known as multiple attachment.

It is thought that our first experience of attachment and bonding provides a 'blueprint' for subsequent relationships. Poor or faulty attachment, or problems with parental bonding, may lead to feelings of insecurity and difficulties in forming and maintaining relationships later in life. As their social and intellectual abilities develop, infants are increasingly able to communicate and interact with other people. This is partly the result of the increasing experience that infants gain of other people and the world around them. However, making friends and playing cooperatively also require some practice. Opportunities to mix and play with other children have a positive effect on the development of an infant's relationship-building skills.

Intellectual development during infancy

Thinking is an intellectual, or cognitive, activity. During early infancy babies tend to respond mainly to physical stimuli. They cry when they are wet, cold and hungry, for example. This is a relatively primitive level of intellectual response. Jean Piaget, a Swiss psychologist who studied and wrote about cognitive development, called infancy the sensorimotor stage of intellectual development. He claimed that infants learn about the world by using their senses (touch, hearing, sight, smell and taste – hence 'sensori') and through physical activity (hence 'motor'). There is very limited cognitive or intellectual activity involved in this type of learning. For example, infants don't deliberately plan or use their memories and experiences in a conscious way.

Thinking skills gradually improve as an infant grows older and experiences intellectual development. For example, by the end of infancy, a child will learn that people and objects continue to exist in the world even when they can't be seen. This is known as object permanence. In contrast, a baby who is less than eight months old won't usually search for a toy that they see being 'hidden' from view in front of them. This is because they haven't usually developed the thinking ability to know that the toy still exists. In fact, it no longer seems to exist at all! An older infant or young child will look for a toy hidden in this way because their intellectual development enables them to work out that objects don't usually stop existing in the world just because they're out of sight.

Table 2 – Intellectual development during infancy

Age	Developmental change
Birth	A baby explores, using their senses to learn
1 month	A baby is able to recognise their parents or main carers by sight and smell
3 months	A baby learns by playing with their hands, holding and grasping objects
6 months	An infant is aware of their parent's or carer's voice and can take part in simple play activities
9 months	An infant recognises familiar toys and pictures, joins in games with familiar people and is able to respond to simple instructions
12 months	An infant can copy other people's behaviour and is able to use objects (e.g. brush or spoon) appropriately
15 months	An infant can remember people, recognise and sort shapes and knows some parts of body ('Where is your nose?')
18 months	An infant is able to recognise themselves in a picture or reflection, can respond to simple instructions and is able to remember and recall simple information
2 years	A child can complete simple jigsaw puzzles and develops a basic understanding of the consequences of their actions
2½ years	A child is now usually very inquisitive, asking lots of questions, knows their own name and can find details in pictures
3 years	A child can usually understand time, is able to recognise different colours, can compare the size of different objects (bigger, smaller) and is able to remember the words to their favourite songs and rhymes

Developing language skills

Learning the basics of a spoken language is an important part of intellectual development during infancy. Babies begin developing communication skills almost straight from birth. Smiles, movements and noises quickly become ways of communicating with caregivers. Babies can also receive information and communicate their feelings from a very early age. Words don't usually become a feature of communication before an infant is one year old. First words are preceded by lots of 'babbling'. Once an older infant begins using words they will quickly develop their vocabulary, putting words into short sentences, and learning a few new words each day.

Social development during infancy

As their social and intellectual abilities develop, infants are increasingly able to communicate and interact with other people. This is partly the result of the increasing experience that an infant gains of other people and the world around them. However, making friends and playing cooperatively also require some practice. Opportunities to mix and play with other children have a positive effect on the development of an infant's relationship-building skills.

See also – Attachment; Autonomy; Piaget, Jean

Further reading

Doherty, J. and Hughes, M. (2013) *Child Development: theory and practice 0–11*. Harlow: Pearson.

Smith, P.K., Cowie, H. and Blades, M. (2015) *Understanding Children's Development*, 6th edition. Chichester: John Wiley & Sons.

Child poverty

In basic terms, this refers to the number of children living in poverty in the UK. This is defined as living in a household with less than half the national average income after deducting housing costs.

Child poverty is an issue and major concern for health and social care professionals because of the effects it has on the development and wellbeing of children. Compared to other western and European countries, the UK has relatively high levels of child poverty. Using figures provided from the government's Department for Work and Pensions, the Child Poverty Action Group (CPAG, 2017) reported that there were 4 million children living in poverty in the UK in 2015–16. That's 30% of children, or 9 in a classroom of 30.

A child's risk of living in poverty increases if:
- they live in a family where no adults are in work
- they live in a large family (3+ children)
- welfare benefits are the main or only source of family income
- the adult wage earners lose their jobs or have their benefits cut.

Obtaining work is no longer a way of avoiding or escaping from poverty in the UK. The Department of Work and Pensions figures show that two-thirds of children in poverty live in a family where at least one member works. This work may be part-time or may be in a low-paid job. Having insufficient money to cope with their circumstances is the fundamental reason for families being in poverty. Not being able to get work, loss of employment, benefit changes and a rise in living costs are all closely associated with families slipping into or being trapped in poverty.

Living in poverty has a damaging effect on a child's development and health during their formative childhood years and also later in life. The CPAG (2017) states that "growing up in poverty means being cold, going hungry, not being able to join in activities with friends". Child poverty is also associated with low birthweight, childhood respiratory diseases, and a higher incidence of obesity, heart disease, mental health problems and diabetes in later life. Children who receive free school meals are 28% less likely to achieve five GCSEs graded A*–C than their more affluent peers.

See also – Child development; Families; Poverty

References and further reading

Child Poverty Action Group (2017) *Child Poverty: facts and figures*. Available at www.cpag.org.uk (accessed 27 March 2018)

Jones, N. and Sumner, A. (2011) *Child Poverty, Evidence and Policy: mainstreaming children in international development*. Bristol: Policy Press.

Citizenship

Citizenship is a status given to individuals who then have legal rights and responsibilities in relation to a specific nation or community. In the twenty-first century, a person's citizenship status is generally given or acquired on the basis of an individual's place of birth or residency. Whilst citizenship is associated with rights and responsibilities, it is also closely associated with heritage, identity and a sense of belonging to a particular place or community.

Sociologist T. H. Marshall (1973) developed a theory of citizenship that saw it as emerging and developing alongside industrialisation, with eighteenth-century civil rights leading to nineteenth-century political rights and then twentieth-century social rights. As such, the concept of citizenship incorporates the idea of:

- civil citizenship – based on property ownership and the rights and obligations to respect other people's rights to property and to maintain social order. However, this left non-property owners without citizenship and political rights.
- political citizenship – based on the extension of voting rights to different sections of the population as well as the right to free association and free speech.
- social citizenship – based on the right to social welfare and the obligation to contribute to the collective provision of welfare and other benefits for those in society who need them.

Critics of Marshall's conception of citizenship point out that whilst he provides a descriptive account of what happened in the evolution of UK citizenship rights, he doesn't explain why the different types of rights were granted in the order or at the historical moments they were. Marshall's approach to citizenship also doesn't anticipate or take into account the development of the European Union, the process of mass migration or refugee crises that have seen large number of people enter the UK and obtain citizenship rights. Marshall's approach also doesn't anticipate the way that social rights can be reversed in times of austerity when welfare spending and entitlement to services are reduced.

Sociologists and political scientists interested in citizenship have argued that environmental citizenship is developing and should be considered as a new set of rights and obligations. This new form of citizenship focuses on the rights of all citizens to expect a safe, clean, sustainable environment as well as obligations not to pollute, damage or harm the natural or human-made environments in which they live. This type of citizenship implies an obligation to protect and maintain the natural environment for future generations.

See also – Community; Globalisation; Industrialisation

Reference and further reading

Lewis, G. (2004) *Citizenship: personal lives and social policy*. Cambridge: Policy Press.
Marshall, T.H. (1973) *Class, Citizenship and Social Development*. Westport, CT: Greenwood Press.

A
B
C
D
E
F
G
H
I
J
K
L
M
N
O
P
Q
R
S
T
U
V
W
X
Y
Z

Classical conditioning

Classical conditioning is a basic, associative learning process that occurs when two stimuli are repeatedly paired. A response that is naturally produced by the first stimulus is eventually elicited by the second, non-naturally occurring stimulus alone.

Ivan Pavlov (1849–1936) first illustrated the process and principles of classical conditioning. In Pavlov's experiments a dog was attached to a harness and to monitors that measured the rate at which it salivated. Pavlov thought that he could learn more about digestion in dogs if he measured the amount of saliva they produced when food was presented to them. However, Pavlov noticed that the dogs used in his experiment didn't have to taste or smell any food to begin salivating. They would salivate as soon as they realised food was being brought to them. For example, the dogs would begin salivating when they heard the footsteps of the approaching experimenter or laboratory assistant. This intrigued Pavlov because the belief at the time was that dogs and other animals salivated as a reflex response to food touching their tongue. Pavlov wondered instead whether the dogs were salivating because they had somehow learnt to associate food with the sound of the experimenter's steps, and that they were salivating in anticipation of the food. Pavlov worked out what was happening and in the process also identified the main principles of associative learning or classical conditioning.

Classical conditioning explained

Food makes a dog salivate automatically – they don't have to think about it or learn to salivate when presented with food. In behavioural terms, this is known as an unconditioned response (UR). The food causing salivation is known as an unconditioned stimulus (US).

Pavlov's experiment involved presenting a dog with food whilst he rang a bell. The aim was to see if the dog would learn to associate the bell with food. Pavlov found that repeated trials of this pairing (bell plus food) led the dog to associate the bell with food. In fact, after a short while the dog would salivate simply when the bell was rung (and no food was presented). Pavlov explained this by saying that the dog had developed or learned a conditioned response (CR) of salivation in response to the conditioned stimulus (CS) of the bell.

In simple terms, Pavlov's experiment demonstrates that animals partly acquire their behaviour through conditioning processes (learning). Humans are animals too, so the principles of associative learning also apply to us! For example, road vehicle drivers have (usually) been conditioned to put their foot on the brake when they see a red traffic light.

See also – Behaviourism; Operant conditioning; Reinforcement

Further reading

Gross, R. (2015) *Psychology: the science of mind and behaviour*, 7th edition. London: Hodder Education.

Clinical iceberg

The concept of the 'clinical iceberg' refers to the large amount of illness and disease within the population that is undiagnosed and unreported.

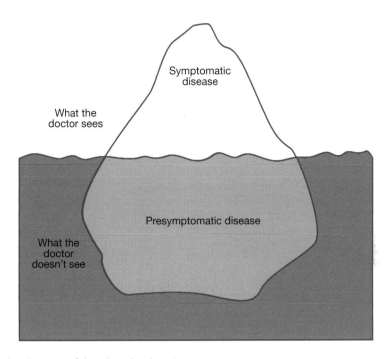

Symptomatic disease

What the doctor sees

Presymptomatic disease

What the doctor doesn't see

Figure 3 – The elements of the 'clinical iceberg'.

Statistics describing patterns of illness and disease are usually compiled from GP consultation or hospital episode data. This data is then used for healthcare commissioning, service planning and policy development purposes. The level of reported illness and diagnosed disease is inevitably an underestimate of the real or actual levels of health problems in the community. Reported illness and disease are the visible part of a much larger clinical iceberg. Below the surface lies the bulk of unreported illness and disease experiences. Social scientists suggest that some health issues such as dementia, mental illness and prostate cancer, for example, are more likely to go unreported because they carry a social stigma. People are more reluctant to consult a doctor in the early, possibly treatable, stages of these conditions or may not have the capacity to recognise they are unwell.

See also – Demography; Epidemiology

Further reading

Somerville, M., Kumaran, K. and Anderson, R. (2016) *Public Health and Epidemiology at a Glance*. Chichester: Wiley Blackwell.

Wilson, F. and Mabhala, M. (2008) *Key Concepts in Public Health*. London: SAGE Publications.

Cognitive perspective

A cognition is a mental action, event or process that involves acquiring knowledge and understanding through thought, experience, and the senses. The cognitive perspective is an approach to psychology that sees cognition as central to human psychological development and functioning.

The cognitive approach is distinctive in the way that it sees human beings as information-processors and compares human mental processes to software running on a computer (the brain).

The cognitive perspective rose to prominence in the late 1950s when it started to challenge the narrow focus that behaviourism had on observable behaviour. Cognitive psychologists believed that internal mental processes should also be studied alongside behaviour. Psychologists and care workers using this perspective now typically study or work with people experiencing perceptual, memory, language and intellectual development or thinking problems – that is, aspects of cognition (mental activity), or the way the brain works.

Many contemporary psychologists would describe themselves as cognitive psychologists. The cognitive approach, and the view that mental events are characterised by an information flow that has to be dealt with, is very popular in health and social care settings too. Specialist counsellors and therapists using forms of cognitive therapy, doctors, nurses and other healthcare practitioners and social care workers also incorporate cognitive techniques into their relationship-building and intervention strategies. All draw on the 'cognitive triad' concept that links thinking, emotion and behaviour but also recognises that the brain's ability to process information is central to this.

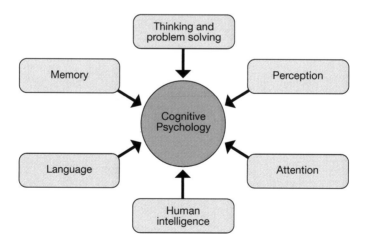

Figure 4 – Key issues in cognitive psychology.

Table 3 – Strengths and weaknesses of cognitive psychology

Strengths	Weaknesses/limitations
Recognises that influences on human behaviour are broader and more complex than simple stimulus-response factors	Ignores the role of biology, emotions, consciousness and free will in human learning and behaviour
Shows how mental processes and the brain play a key part in the way people learn and behave	Doesn't recognise the role of the unconscious and early experiences in understanding an individual's behaviour
Sees the person as making some active choices (through creating meaning, memory, decision-making and use of judgement) in what they learn and how they behave	Ignores the human experience of emotions and the powerful ways they can affect learning, behaviour and development
Cognitive behavioural therapy (CBT) is based on a scientific, evidence-based approach to psychological treatment	CBT is criticised for treating a person's symptoms rather than the causes of their problems
The cognitive approach can be applied quite widely in the health and social care field	It is reductionist and deterministic, suggesting that complex human psychological processes and experiences can be explained largely in terms of brain functioning

See also – Cognitive behavioural therapy; Depression; Learning difficulties; Piaget, Jean; Post-traumatic stress disorder

Further reading

Fairholm, I. (2012) *Issues, Debates and Approaches in Psychology*. Basingstoke: Palgrave.
Gross, R. (2015) *Psychology: the science of mind and behaviour*, 7th edition. London: Hodder Education.

Cognitive behavioural therapy

Cognitive behavioural therapy is a form of talking therapy that helps people to change the way they think and behave as a way of managing their problems. It is based on the premise that cognition (acquiring knowledge and forming beliefs) has a direct influence on a person's mood and behaviour.

Cognitive behavioural therapy (CBT) was developed by Aaron T. Beck (1967) to treat depression. Beck identified a 'cognitive triad' (see *Figure 5*) based on a negative self-appraisal that leads to negative beliefs about the world and the future – the individual sees themselves as powerless to overcome their difficulties.

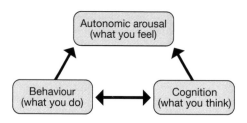

Figure 5 – The ABC of CBT theory.

The aim of CBT is to challenge negative thoughts and to enable each person to develop an alternative, positive view of the world. A 'thought diary' may be used to collect or catch 'negative automatic thoughts' and patterns of negative thinking. The care practitioner and client can then work out ways of challenging them. A key strategy is to consider the evidence for the negative thoughts and what the alternatives might be.

Cognitive behavioural therapy is widely used in UK health and social care services. It is an effective treatment for anxiety and depression and is often available within primary care and mental health services. In practice, CBT is easy to engage with and provides a short-term, evidence-based form of mental health treatment that can be delivered by a range of health and social care workers who have received additional training. It also has the advantage of turning a person from a 'patient' into their own therapist. This is because, once some new coping strategies have been learnt, CBT enables the individual to identify and deal with their own thinking errors.

See also – Anxiety; Behaviour; Challenging behaviour; Cognitive perspective; Depression; Mental illness; Phobias; Post-traumatic stress disorder

Reference and further reading

Beck, A.T. (1967) *The Diagnosis and Management of Depression*. Philadelphia, PA: University of Pennsylvania Press.

Simmons, J. and Griffiths, R. (2017) *CBT for Beginners*, 3rd edition. London: SAGE Publications.

Cognitive development

Cognitive development focuses on the human ability to think and to understand the mental processes that lie behind this ability and the part the brain plays in these processes.

The term *cognition* comes from the Greek word for 'knowing'. Cognitive psychologists believe that behaviour is based on knowing about the situation in which the behaviour occurs. As a result, cognitive theories of development encourage parents and teachers to help children think about what they're doing, thereby appealing to curiosity and interest. *Figure 6* summarises the main elements of the cognitive development process.

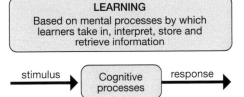

LEARNING
Based on mental processes by which learners take in, interpret, store and retrieve information

stimulus → Cognitive processes → response

Figure 6 – Cognitive development is concerned with thinking and understanding skills.

Cognitive theories of development arose in part to explain how learning involved more than just behavioural reinforcement. Research into how monkeys learn suggested that motivation to learn isn't only induced by the anticipation of a reward, but also by enjoying the learning process itself.

In one study, reported by David Wood (1998), a monkey was being conditioned to pull a lever that sometimes delivered a reinforcer in the form of a peanut. However, when the peanut arrived, the monkey often stored it in its food pouch inside the mouth. As the experiment proceeded, the monkey's food pouch bulged to capacity. But, despite being unlikely to gain from further 'reinforcement', the monkey continued operating the lever. It seemed that the monkey wasn't carrying on with the lever operations to win a reward, but because it found the task interesting!

Cognitive development affects a range of mental, or brain-driven, skills and abilities. These include:

- language acquisition and use
- thinking and problem-solving skills
- attention and focusing
- perception
- memory (storage and recall)
- human intelligence.

A focus on cognitive development and the basic idea that information-processing and cognition are fundamentally *human* experiences are central to the cognitive perspective within psychology. Problems and difficulties with cognitive development are an important feature of learning disability and specific learning difficulties.

See also – Child development; Cognitive perspective; Piaget, Jean

Reference and further reading

Keenan, T., Evans, S. and Crowley, K. (2016) *An Introduction to Child Development*, 3rd edition. London: SAGE Publications.

Wood, D. (1998) *How Children Think and Learn*, 2nd edition. Oxford: Blackwell.

Cognitive dissonance

Cognitive dissonance is a psychological concept that captures the sense of mental stress and the feelings of discomfort that a person experiences when they:
- hold two or more contradictory beliefs, values or thoughts simultaneously
- behave in a way that contradicts their beliefs and values
- are faced with new information that conflicts with their existing knowledge, beliefs or values.

Leon Festinger (1958), an American psychologist, is most closely associated with the concept of cognitive development. Festinger's cognitive dissonance theory focuses on how humans strive for internal consistency in their attitudes, values and beliefs and what happens when we experience psychological inconsistency. The way to reduce cognitive dissonance is to change behaviour or to change your attitudes, values or beliefs. The goal of doing this is to reduce psychological tension and distress. Festinger (1958) argues that dissonance reduction can be achieved by:
- changing a behaviour or cognition ('I'll stop eating ice cream')
- justifying/rationalising the behaviour or conflicting cognition ('It's OK to eat just this one ice cream')
- justifying the behaviour or cognition by adding a new legitimising cognition ('I can eat ice cream if I go to the gym more often')
- trying to ignore or deny any information that conflicts with existing beliefs ('Ice cream isn't that high in fat anyway').

Adjustments between conflicting cognitions or between a cognition and conflicting behaviour can result in:
- a consonant relationship – realigning cognitions or a cognition and behaviour
- an irrelevant relationship – breaking the link between cognitions or a cognition and behaviour ('I'd love a doughnut, but I'll brush my hair instead')
- a dissonant relationship – preserving conflicting cognitions or a cognition and behaviour that is contradictory.

Cognitive dissonance remains a useful psychological concept as it helps to explain why people change their attitudes and behaviour and can be used to promote healthy and positive social behaviours.

See also – Attitudes; Cognitive behaviour therapy; Cognitive development

Reference and further reading

Festinger, L. (1957) *A Theory of Cognitive Dissonance*. Stanford, CA: Stanford University Press.
Gross, R. (2015) *Psychology: the science of mind and behaviour*, 7th edition. London: Hodder Education.

Community

Community is a contested, shifting construct in social science that has been used in different ways. In basic terms, it refers to a group of people living in a particular place or geographical location (territorial communities) or to a group of people with shared interests or a common identity who interact with each other regularly and for specific purposes (communities of interest). It is concerned with a set of social relationships that occur within certain boundaries.

The term community has a long history in the social sciences. In the feudal era it was used to distinguish 'common people' from those of rank, but gradually came to describe people living in a particular area or who shared particular interests. In the nineteenth century, Ferdinand Tönnies, one of the early pioneers of sociological theory, identified communities as cohesive social entities that exist within a broader society. He contrasted *Gemeinschaft* (community bonds) with *Gesellschaft* (associational bonds) and felt the former was in decline as a result of industrialisation and urbanisation during the nineteenth century. Social changes, particularly industrialisation and the shift to modern society, were also seen by Émile Durkheim to be a key factor in changing traditional sources of community solidarity in the nineteenth century.

Notions of community based on the idea of a bounded territory have a long history in sociological research and discussion. Many community studies, such as Wilmott and Young's (1969) classic study *Family and Kinship in East London*, were carried out in the 1950s and 1960s, for example. These studies tended to look inwards, focusing on detailed patterns of social relations within the community. Their weakness was that they usually failed to consider or show how the lives of people within a bounded community were connected to the world outside of it. Additionally, they contributed to what is now a stereotypical view of 'community' as a nostalgic place where friends and neighbours meet and interact with each other, where there are accessible and useful services as well as a pervading sense of support and wellbeing ('community spirit') shared by all. Global migration as well as increased movement of people within the UK over the last half century has unsettled this idea of bounded communities. It has led sociologists to focus more on the way 'communities' can exist across geographical boundaries, through dispersed social networks of mobile and migrant workers, and in other non-geographical forms.

Sociological critics of the 'bounded community' concept have shifted their focus to the more flexible idea of people experiencing 'community' through a 'community of interest'. This definition of 'community' is typically associated with feelings of belonging and identification, shared beliefs, interests or common occupations. As a result, it is now common to hear people speak of the 'Muslim community', the 'gay community' or the 'academic community', for example. The concept of community of interests allows sociologists to consider how communities are formed and maintained across national and international territorial boundaries.

Social scientists question both the stereotypical view of community and the notion that there is no longer any community solidarity in society. They also point out that there are many different types of community in society, some of which are not positive (e.g. criminal communities, drug-taking communities, paedophile communities, etc.), and that a community may include some people whilst excluding others or may be experienced as supportive by some but stifling by others. For some people, community is found and experienced at work rather than where they live. For others, social and leisure activities carried out with a group of like-minded people, either in person or in a virtual online setting, provide them with an experience of community. As a result, it's important to note that within social science, community carries multiple meanings and can be conceptualised and experienced in a variety of ways.

See also – Ethnicity; Gender; Globalisation; Identity; Migration

Reference and further reading

Calhoun, C. (2018) *Community – Key Concepts*. Cambridge: Polity Press.
Young, M. and Wilmott, M. (1969) *Family and Kinship in East London*. Harmondsworth: Pelican.

Conformity

Conformity is a concept that plays an important part in the psychology of social influence. It refers to the factors and processes that influence people to follow (or conform to) the behaviour of others.

Conformity is quite a big topic within the psychology of social influence. Majority and minority influence are two key aspects of it. Majority influence refers to situations where people follow the group, whilst minority influence refers to situations where people are influenced by and follow the minority. A number of theories have been developed to explain both majority and minority influence. Deutsch and Gerard (1955) identified two types of majority influence:

- Normative influence – where, at least publicly, the person is motivated to fit in so they are liked and accepted by others. In private the person may disagree with the majority but doesn't reveal this publicly.
- Informational influence – where a person who is self-conscious, unsure or worried about getting something wrong follows others whom they believe do know what to do. A person in this situation will conform publicly and privately.

The psychology of social influence has been important in showing how and why people tend to conform to group influences, particularly in situations of uncertainty. Asch's (1951) 'line experiment' showed how people are frequently influenced by others in their judgement even when the evidence in front of them indicates that the group is wrong. Majority influence is typically too powerful for an individual to resist.

The existence of minority influence shows that it is possible to influence the group from a minority position. Moscovici *et al.* (1969) argued that the minority needed to be forceful, persistent and unwavering whilst also appearing flexible and open-minded. If the minority maintain a consistent position or approach and also have a strong person investment in what they are doing or saying, they are more likely to influence others. Where minority influence is effective it tends to follow a 'snowball' pattern. That is, support for the minority position will be small at first but will gradually grow as more people start to agree, until a level of momentum is reached that leads to the minority position becoming the majority one.

See also – Authority; Obedience

References

Asch, E.E. (1951) 'Effect of group pressure upon the modification and distortion of judgements'. In H. Guetzkow (ed.), *Groups, Leadership and Men*. Pittsburgh, PA: Carnegie Press.

Deutsch, M. and Gerard, H.B. (1955) A study of normative and informational social influence upon individual judgements. *Journal of Abnormal and Social Psychology*, **51:** 629–636.

Moscovici, S., Lage, E. and Naffrechoux, M. (1969) Influence of a consistent minority on the responses of a majority in a color perception task. *Sociometry*, **32:** 365–380.

Consumerism/consumption

> Consumerism refers to a lifestyle that involves the continual purchasing and consumption of goods for personal fulfilment.

Consumerism and consumption have been the focus of sociologists since the early days of sociology in the nineteenth century. This was partly triggered by an increase in the production of material goods that followed the Industrial Revolution in the UK. Initial consumption of consumer goods by the upper classes and aristocracy was followed by the gradual spread of consumerism to other social groups from the mid-nineteenth century onwards. Mass consumption of goods and the consumer lifestyle were established as a way of life by the mid-twentieth century in western and developed economies. Consumerism is now associated with relatively affluent societies, though consumption pressures and practices can affect all social groups within a capitalist society, regardless of whether they are rich or poor.

Sociologists who study consumption argue that many developed societies are now economically dependent on mass consumerism. One of the problems with this is that mass consumerism relies on the easy availability of credit. This can result in people living with large amounts of personal debt and an economy that becomes dependent on ever increasing but ultimately unsustainable levels of credit to support 'normal' and expected patterns of consumption. Sociologists concerned with the development of a consumer society tend to focus on the impact that consumerism can have on identity formation, the striving for status (achieved through purchasing and consuming certain commodities) that affects social relations and broader concerns with the environmental impact of high consumption levels on the natural environment.

From a psychological perspective, consumerism works by turning desires or 'wants' into needs. Through advertising and marketing, people are encouraged to realise their desires by meeting what they see as their needs. Critics of consumerism argue that conflating wants and needs and convincing people they must, ought to or deserve to buy, own or consume a particular product amounts to deception. In particular, critics argue that consumerism is based on false beliefs that consuming certain products or brands increases a person's chance of experiencing happiness and self-fulfilment.

See also – Alienation; Capitalism; Globalisation; Identity; Ideology; Industrialisation; Power; Status

Further reading

Haralambos, M. and Holborn, M. (2013) *Sociology Themes and Perspectives*, 8th edition. London: Collins Education.

Stearns, P.N. (2006) *Consumerism in World History: the global transformation of desire*, 2nd edition. Abingdon: Routledge.

Culture

Culture is a complex, contested concept widely used in the social sciences. Prominent amongst its various meanings is that it refers to the way of life that characterises a society or social group.

Culture is seen in various ways as something that is essential to, and an inevitable part of, any society. It is a concept that holds notions of shared attitudes, values and beliefs and characteristic ways of life. In sociological terms, culture is what binds people together as a collectivity in a society. It is a thing that we share and a 'more-than-the sum-of-the-parts' aspect of the human world that enables us to make human activities and relationships 'meaningful'.

Sensitivity to culture is an important feature of 'sociological thinking' because:
- it helps us to distinguish between the social and natural aspects of human life
- it enables us to identify and acknowledge the existence of social diversity within a society and between different societies
- it allows us to challenge the notion that some social groups and ways of life are 'superior' to others.

A sensitivity to culture and cultural difference allows us to identify, accommodate and respond respectfully to the culturally specific forms that societies and social behaviours take. One consequence of this for healthcare workers is that we need to develop and apply an awareness of culturally diverse ways of help-seeking and illness behaviour in order to meet the needs of all service users in a culturally diverse population.

Culture, health and development

Culture may affect physical growth and development where cultural beliefs or practices influence food choices, patterns of exercise and use of healthcare services, for example. Social development may also be affected by culture where cultural beliefs or practices influence attitudes, values and opportunities to develop and experience friendships and other non-family relationships. Emotional development may also be affected by extended family structures, by the closeness or expected pattern of relationships within the family and by a person's identification with their cultural heritage. In these different ways, culture can play a very important, though often unseen, role in shaping our personal growth and development.

It is also important to note that the psychological approaches and theories we use – our ways of understanding and explaining psychological development – may not be universally applicable. Cross-cultural variations exist in the way people develop and experience themselves and the world psychologically. It is important that care workers are not culturally 'blind' to the influence a person's cultural background may have on their behaviour and way of relating to others.

See also – Discourse; Ethnicity; Gender; Power; Society; Status

Further reading

Alexander, J.C. and Thompson, K. (2017) *A Contemporary Introduction to Sociology: culture and society in transition,* 3rd edition. Abingdon: Routledge.

Haralambos, M. and Holborn, M. (2013) *Sociology Themes and Perspectives*, 8th edition. London: Collins Education.

Data

The term data simply refers to items of information (variables) that are collected together or produced for reference or analysis.

Data plays a fundamental part in social science. Social scientists obtain data from primary and secondary sources. Primary data is new, original information collected directly by a researcher undertaking a research investigation. Secondary data is pre-existing information that a researcher hasn't collected personally but which they reuse in their own research investigation. Secondary data can be thought of as a second-hand report or record. A social science-based research study may make use of both primary and secondary data.

Within social science, data is often described as being either quantitative or qualitative. Researchers who set out to collect data that measures how many, how often, what percentage or proportion or 'To what extent is there a connection between X and Y?' are seeking quantitative data. Social science research that is based on quantitative data always involves measuring in some way. The chief characteristic of quantitative data is that it is numerical – or can be reduced to numerical items of information. When quantitative data has been collected, statistical techniques are used to establish and describe the numerical patterns and relationships that exist in the data. Social scientists will often then visualise their quantitative data using graphs, images, models or other visual analysis tools.

Not all data is reducible to a numerical form and researchers don't always want to collect measurements of things. For example, a lot of healthcare research is conducted into people's experiences. This produces non-numerical qualitative data. Researchers who use a naturalistic approach to investigate people's feelings and beliefs, or ways of life, find qualitative data in a variety of sources and are interested in appreciating the meanings attached to them. Research investigations that are primarily seeking these non-numerical forms of data are often called qualitative studies.

Healthcare workers make use of both primary and secondary data in their clinical practice. For example, recording an individual's pulse, blood pressure and respirations will generate primary data. This may be analysed and compared to standardised tables of normal pulse, blood pressure or respiration rates, which is secondary data. Scans, laboratory results, test responses and a person's own account of their health and illness experiences, their pain levels or their felt symptoms all provide secondary data that practitioners must incorporate into their clinical judgements.

See also – Demography; Research methods

Further reading

Ellis, P. (2016) *Understanding Research for Nursing Students*, 3rd edition. London: Learning Matters.

Lindsay, B. (2007) *Understanding Research and Evidence-Based Practice*. Exeter: Reflect Press.

Defence mechanisms

> In psychodynamic theory, defence mechanisms are coping strategies designed to reduce anxiety that arises from unacceptable or harmful impulses deep in the unconscious.

Psychodynamic psychologists argue that people often use defence mechanisms to try to control their anxieties without being aware that they are doing so. Their anxieties may then manifest themselves in physical symptoms and illnesses, challenging behaviour or emotional distress. This can be very difficult for both the individuals concerned and healthcare staff to deal with – the person has some physical symptoms or problems but there is no obvious physical, medical or other cause.

In circumstances like these, particularly where the symptoms have been long-lasting, a psychodynamic approach can be helpful in revealing the psychological root causes of the person's problems, and also provides a way of addressing them.

Within the psychodynamic perspective, defence mechanisms are a way of protecting the ego from distress. They allow us to unconsciously block out experiences that overwhelm us. *Table 4* describes a range of examples of defence mechanisms.

Table 4 – Examples of ego defence mechanisms

Defence mechanism	Effect	Example
Repression	Person forgets an event or experience	No recollection of a serious car crash
Regression	Revert to an earlier stage of development	Bedwetting when sibling is born or school begins
Denial	Pushing events or emotion out of consciousness	Refusal to accept you have a substance misuse problem
Projection	Personal faults or negative feelings are attributed to someone else	Accusing a colleague of being angry or thoughtless when you are really feeling this way
Displacement	Redirecting desire or other strong emotions onto another person	Shouting at your partner instead of at yourself or your best friend

See also – Freud; Psychoanalysis; Psychodynamic perspective; Unconscious mind

Further reading

Gross, R. (2015) *Psychology: the science of mind and behaviour*, 7th edition. London: Hodder Education.

Demography

Demography involves the statistical study of the health experiences and social characteristics of a human population.

Demographers compile a range of different statistics from the size of national populations to the composition (by age, ethnicity, gender, social class, etc.) of regions and communities. Demographic profiles are widely used by central and local government planners to plan for infrastructure and service provision (health, education, criminal justice, welfare payments, etc.) across the country. Similarly, demographers carry out detailed statistical analysis of the national census (carried out every ten years) and other statistics, such as migration, fertility, mortality and hospital episode data, to adapt service provision and government intervention in relation to changes in the size and composition of the population.

Demographic data is used by social scientists to understand the composition of society (according to class, gender, ethnicity, etc.) and the changing nature of social relations. For example, the incidence of marriage, divorce/separation and cohabitation, as well as when and within what kind of relationships women have children, can reveal a lot about intimacy, families and the stability of households in contemporary society. Social scientists use this kind of data as the trigger for research studies, as a quantitative evidence base on which to develop their analyses and understanding of social life and as a way of contextualising social changes and comparing their own findings against the bigger, comparative picture of society as a whole.

See also – Age; Data; Epidemiology; Ethnicity; Families; Gender; Social class

Further reading

Dorling, D. and Gietel-Basten, S. (2018) *Why Demography Matters*. Cambridge: Polity Press.

Depression

Depression is a psychiatric diagnosis associated with persistently low mood accompanied by other symptoms of physical, psychological and social disturbance.

A person is likely to be diagnosed with depression if they have experienced five of the following symptoms over a two-week period:

- Feeling low or depressed most of the time
- Significant weight loss
- Sleep disturbance (insomnia or early waking)
- Fatigue
- Guilt feelings
- Feelings of hopelessness
- Poor concentration
- Intrusive and disrupted thinking.

The biomedical approach to depression identifies biological causes (e.g. low levels of the neurotransmitters serotonin, noradrenaline and dopamine). Psychological approaches identify cognitive distortions (e.g. negative thinking) and learned helplessness. Social approaches suggest that traumatic life events, such as abuse during childhood or a later developmental stage, social isolation and lack of social support may also trigger or sustain depression. Treatment for depression is typically a response to the apparent cause: antidepressant medication to act on neurotransmitters; talking therapies to address cognitive distortions; and befriending, social support and activity-based interventions to address social isolation.

Social scientists have focused on a number of aspects of the diagnosis of depression, on the process of becoming 'depressed' and on the way in which people experience depression. The fuzzy boundary between 'sadness' as a normal human experience and depression as a pathological mood disorder (an abnormal human experience) has led some social scientists to suggest that normal sadness has been medicalised over the last century (Horwitz and Wakefield, 2007). Whilst being sad seems to be a universal emotional state, the way in which it is understood and explained as 'depression' is not. Different cultures vary in the way they understand, explain and respond to sadness. Even in western psychiatry, depression is defined in different ways: some psychiatrists focus on mood disturbance whilst others focus on cognitive distortions. Similarly, sociologists have noted that depression is more likely to be diagnosed in women than men (Mental Health Foundation, 2013). Explanations for this include 'gendered' diagnosis resulting from 'sex stereotypes' that assume female emotional fragility as well as the effects of gender socialisation that make it easier for women to identify, talk about and seek help for emotional and psychological problems.

See also – Biomedical model; Labelling theory; Psychiatry; Psychological perspectives

References

Horwitz, A.V. and Wakefield, J.C. (2007) *The Loss of Sadness: how psychiatry transformed normal sorrow into depressive disorder*. New York: Oxford University Press.
Mental Health Foundation (2013) *Mental Health Statistics*. Available at www.mentalhealth.org.uk (accessed 27 March 2018)

Developmental norms

Developmental norms are the milestones or stages of physical, emotional or cognitive development that human beings are expected to achieve or follow at particular ages.

Human growth and development follows a predictable pattern. Observation, experience and research have shown that specific patterns of growth and development tend to occur within particular time periods. Growth and developmental changes also tend to occur in a particular sequence. For example, when a baby can sit up unaided, it will develop the ability to crawl, followed by the ability to stand up and then the ability to walk. A 'developmental norm' is created by linking this sequence of expected growth and development to an expected timeframe. Knowledge of developmental norms provides a useful guide for assessing an infant's or a child's pattern of growth and development.

A skilled, knowledgeable practitioner would be able to use their understanding of developmental norms to identify whether an individual's development at specific points was age-appropriate. They would also be able to identify developmental delay and problems. Various cognitive and social skills are assessed as well as physical and motor abilities.

The value of developmental norms is that they can provide health and social care workers with hard data (based on scientific theory and observation) about an individual's development relative to that of others. Identification of developmental problems can then quickly lead to treatment or other interventions to support the child or young person. It is important to note that the times at which different individuals achieve the same developmental norms may vary. It is not correct to say an infant, child or adolescent is 'abnormal' if they reach a developmental norm at a slightly different time from the expected pattern. There may be a number of reasons for advanced and delayed development, none of which make the individual's development 'abnormal'.

See also – Attachment; Child development; Genetics

Further reading

Doherty, J. and Hughes, M. (2013) *Child Development: theory and practice 0–11.* Harlow: Pearson.

Smith, P.K., Cowie, H. and Blades, M. (2015) *Understanding Children's Development,* 6th edition. Chichester: John Wiley & Sons.

Disabilities

'Disability' is a contested concept in social science. It is associated with a lack of capacity or ability that affects an individual's functioning.

The Disability Discrimination Act (1995) describes a disabled person as:

"anyone with a physical or mental impairment which has a substantial and long-term adverse effect upon their ability to carry out normal day to day activities."

This type of medical or 'personal tragedy' definition is typically disputed and rejected by social scientists and disability rights activists. It is contested because it conflates (collapses together) the concepts of *impairment* and *disability*. The DDA (1995) definition suggests that impairment creates, or at least results in, disability. Consequently, Goodley (2010) argues, definitions such as this one suggest disabled people need to find ways of adjusting to *their* disability and that disability is an individual-level problem.

By contrast, social scientists tend to use 'disability' in qualified and specific ways, often making a distinction between dis-ability and the term impairment, or clarifying that they see disability as a socially-determined state that limits an individual's participation in personal, social or work-related activities. Disability, for social scientists, is produced in the interactions between individuals and environmental factors (built environment, social attitudes, lack of support, etc.) and is not located within the person. Using this type of social model of disability, social scientists argue that the causes of disability are located within society and the way it is organised for people with a particular range of abilities.

The way language and terminology are used is important in the 'disability' field because it defines, or sets out, possibilities. The struggle over how to define disability is not just about finding the correct words. It really is a political struggle, an issue to do with how the meaning of 'disability' and the language we use can empower or diminish the people that they refer to. Disability is a term that has negative connotations in British society. Robert Drake (1999) suggests that it conjures up images of the 'paraphernalia of disability', such as wheelchairs, white sticks and charity boxes. Disabled people are often seen as a group who are in constant need of medical help.

Despite seeing them as whole and capable individuals, those who adopt the social model also refer to people who have various forms of impairment as *disabled people*. The term is used to acknowledge the regular, and sometimes continuous, experience that is endured by people who have some form of impairment – one of being excluded from, and frustrated and undermined by the physical environment and social attitudes of the world in which they live. In the medical model, the onus is on the disabled person to adapt to society – not vice versa. The disabled person is encouraged to 'make the best' of his or her situation, and to accept his or her limitations. In the social model, the onus is reversed. Society is seen as having a responsibility to adapt to and accommodate the needs of people who have impairments. The social model does not see impairment as a 'personal tragedy', or disabled people as somehow lesser human beings than 'able-bodied' people.

See also – Biomedical model; Social constructionism; Social model of health

References

Drake, R. (1999) *Understanding Disability Policies*. Basingstoke: Palgrave.

Goodley, D. (2010) *Disability Studies: an interdisciplinary introduction*. London: SAGE Publications.

Discourse

A discourse is a way of thinking or talking about something (e.g. 'health') using a language that makes a particular type of sense (e.g. 'scientific') of the subject, creates knowledge and which shapes a person's behaviour or actions in relation to it.

In its broadest sense, discourse refers to a form of communication, written or spoken. Social scientists argue that such communication is not 'neutral', passive or merely descriptive. Instead, it is argued that discourse (acts of communication) actively shapes a person's knowledge of the world. The term discourse is now widely used within sociological literature to refer to a way of thinking or a set of related statements or events that define relationships between elements of the social world. Michel Foucault, a French philosopher, pioneered the use of discourse within the social sciences by showing how discourse is linked to social structures and social relations – particularly the ways of the powerful. Social scientists have made considerable use of this concept ever since!

One of the key points that social scientists make about discourse is that the particular ways in which we use language have consequences. In essence, our use of language constructs 'reality' in a particular way. So, when we discuss the people nurses work with as 'patients', 'service users' or 'clients' or whether we refer to a regular accident and emergency visitor's problems as 'hypochondria', 'unexplained medical symptoms' or 'attention-seeking', our understanding and response is likely to differ because of the discursive language used.

Sociologists point out that the way language is used to frame our own and other people's experiences controls the way an issue can be discussed. In fact, language makes some issues, experiences and ideas visible and available for discussion whilst also excluding others by denying them a discursive framework. Discussions of 'health' in UK society, for example, are structured and use the language of biomedicine to the extent that biomedical ideas about health, illness and disease are accepted as a normal, common sense part of everyday life. Using religious or spiritual ideas to identify and discuss health concerns now seems illogical, unintelligible and even a sign of mental ill health in mainstream healthcare services. For people born and socialised into contemporary western societies such as the UK, biomedical ideas about health have been integrated into their sense of self and their core beliefs about the world and the way it operates. The language of biomedicine can be said to construct the reality of 'health' and 'illness' for many people.

Discourse remains a useful and productive concept in the social sciences, in that it draws attention to the close links between the creation of knowledge and the operation of discursive power. It also encourages social scientists and practitioners in fields such as healthcare to pay attention to the narratives of disadvantaged, minority or excluded individuals or communities, in order to understand both how dominant discourse works and how it can provide only a partial account of social experiences – often denying, excluding or silencing alternative discourses.

See also – Agency; Anti-psychiatry; Biomedical model; Mental illness; Reflexivity; Self

Further reading

Haralambos, M. and Holborn, M. (2013) *Sociology Themes and Perspectives*, 8th edition. London: Collins Education.

Discrimination

Discrimination is typically used to refer to the less favourable, unjust or unfair treatment of an individual, group or community of people on the basis of their age, gender, ethnicity or sexuality, for example.

A
B
C
D
E
F
G
H
I
J
K
L
M
N
O
P
Q
R
S
T
U
V
W
X
Y
Z

The term discrimination can be used in a number of ways. For example, discrimination involves recognising and understanding the difference between one thing and another, such as when we discriminate between right and wrong or good and bad. This isn't the way in which health and social care workers tend to use or understand this term. This is because discrimination – or more precisely unfair discrimination – also refers to the unjust and unfair treatment of different categories of people because of their race, age, gender or sexuality, for example.

Unfair discrimination can be expressed and experienced in a number of different ways:

- Direct discrimination involves deliberately treating one person less favourably than another and can be an overt abuse of power. The motive or intention behind such treatment is irrelevant. For example, unlawful direct discrimination would occur if a residential home refused to admit a disabled black person as a resident simply because she was black. It is also unlawful for residential homes to set quotas admitting people of different ethnic origins or to reserve places on a racial basis, as this would lead to direct discrimination.
- Indirect discrimination, or the covert use of power, can also occur, for example, where a residential home sets a requirement or condition that when applied equally, disadvantages some social groups because they are less able to satisfy it. Because the condition or requirement works to the detriment of some social groups (and to the advantage of others) it indirectly discriminates against them.

Unfair discrimination doesn't just occur at an individual, interpersonal level. Institutions, including care organisations, have also been accused of operating in ways that discriminate unfairly. Institutional discrimination is usually associated with indirect forms of discrimination. This can occur, for example, where the policies or procedures of a care organisation disadvantage a particular social group whose members are less able to comply with it. Because care organisations are generally keen to promote open and equal access for everyone in their local communities, they now tend to take a positive approach towards identifying and tackling situations that may lead to indirect discrimination.

Unfair discrimination that is obvious and deliberate is known as overt discrimination. Unfair discrimination that happens inadvertently or which is carried out in a secretive, hidden way is known as covert discrimination. Acknowledging diversity and challenging prejudices and all forms of unfair discrimination are important elements of anti-discriminatory practice in care work.

Discrimination is an important issue that affects many people who use and provide health and social care services.

Table 5 – Examples of unfair discrimination

Type of discrimination	What does this involve?
Racism	Unfair discrimination against people because of their 'race' or ethnicity. It can be expressed as: • institutional racism where an organisation inadvertently disadvantages or deliberately treats people of one particular ethnic group less favourably • directly as overt racism • indirectly as covert or inadvertent racism Minority ethnic groups are more likely to experience racism than members of the white majority group in the UK
Sexism	Unfair discrimination against people because of their sex or gender. Sexism: • can occur at institutional, group or an individual level • may be direct and overt or indirect, inadvertent and covert Women are more likely to experience sexism in the UK; the consequences can be fewer opportunities, lack of recognition and unequal pay compared to men, for example
Homophobia	This is the fear and hatred of people who are homosexual and their homosexuality. Homophobia is a prejudice that can lead to: • hostility and unfair discrimination • hate crimes • physical threats and violence People who are homophobic often feel that heterosexuality is 'normal' and that homosexuality somehow presents a threat to normal social order

See also – Diversity; Equalities; Ethics

Further reading

Cuthbert, S. and Quallington, J. (2017) *Values and Ethics for Care Practice*. Banbury: Lantern Publishing.

Thornicroft, G. (2006) *Shunned: discrimination against people with mental illness*. Oxford: Oxford University Press.

Diversity

> Diversity refers to the social, cultural or ethnic differences in the characteristics of individuals within a population.

Diversity is a feature of modern life. The UK has a population that is diverse in many ways. That is, the population consists of people who have a range of different characteristics, needs, beliefs and values. Diversity within the UK population can be understood in terms of:

- 'race'/ethnicity
- culture
- gender
- social class
- sexuality
- disability
- age.

All of these social and cultural differences affect people's needs and have important implications for care practitioners and for care organisations. In particular, health and social care practice needs to acknowledge, respect and accommodate this diversity. Care organisations and practitioners have to meet the particular needs of people of different ages, different genders, people who have differing ethnic and cultural backgrounds and people with a broad range of abilities, disabilities, illnesses and impairments whilst also ensuring people are treated equally. Health and social care workers need to understand the benefits of social and cultural diversity in order to provide appropriate care services in a fair and equal way.

Diversity is not celebrated by everyone in the UK and is a source of fear and resentment for some people who believe they are being 'pushed out' or 'taken over' by 'outsiders'. This can then lead to unfair treatment or unfair discrimination against those who are different from the majority.

See also – Culture; Discrimination; Equalities

Further reading

Patel, J. and Yafai, G. (2016) *Demystifying Diversity: a handbook to navigate equality, diversity and inclusion.* London: Gilgamesh Publishing.

Thompson, N. (2016) *Anti-Discriminatory Practice: equality, diversity and social justice,* 6th edition. London: Palgrave.

Division of labour

Division of labour is a concept that describes the deliberate separation of work tasks and occupations to promote efficiency in a production or work process.

Division of labour is generally thought of as a sociological concept but it has its origins in the work of Adam Smith (1776/1991), an eighteenth-century economist. Smith's observations of the division of labour in a pin-making factory made him realise that breaking down the tasks involved in the production of pins and getting different people to do only one part of the process in a planned, repetitive way led to a big increase in pin production. Sociologist Émile Durkheim (1893/1984) subsequently noted that the industrial division of labour was affecting social relations, particularly social solidarity, in society generally. He argued that within capitalist society, the processes of industrialisation and urbanisation were changing the way people lived their lives and were connected to each other. Durkheim argued that traditional forms of 'mechanical solidarity' resulting from a relatively stable, shared lifestyle where people were deferential to authority and bound to others at a collective level were breaking down. They were being replaced by a new form of 'organic solidarity' in which greater individualism and the division of labour was leading to social solidarity developing in larger, more mutually dependent communities. In effect, the increasing division of labour was making people more reliant on each other and less self-sufficient and isolated.

There is a now complex division of labour in contemporary societies. We are all dependent on others when it comes to meeting our basic needs and sustaining our lifestyles. Few people grow their own food, make their own clothes or build their own houses. In most areas of work, it is also possible to find specialised occupations. This has become the normal, everyday experience of most workers. They just do one part of a more complex process that involves many other people. In the past more people undertook apprenticeships, learnt crafts and became skilled artisans, controlling their own work and making products or providing services from start to finish. Industrialisation and the mechanisation of the workplace eliminated much of the need for skilled artisans and trained professionals. Goods and services could be provided more quickly, cheaply and efficiently through a division of labour. This has had the additional effect of deskilling and disempowering artisans and highly trained practitioners. Critics of the division of labour argue that autonomy has been lost, alienation has increased and work has been degraded as a result.

The concept of division of labour has also been developed by feminist social scientists to explore the gendered nature of the sexual division of labour in society. It was initially used in the 1970s to define and describe the way in which unpaid work and responsibilities in the home were gendered. Women's unpaid labour in the home was contrasted with men's paid work in the labour market. Additionally, feminist sociologists argued that this situation undermined women's job opportunities and status in the workplace and also impacted the types of work they had access to (particularly 'caring' work). More recent research into the distribution of domestic responsibilities within the home has found that a sexual division of labour remains in place. Women still perform the bulk of domestic chores and bear greater childcare responsibilities than men, even when they are also in paid work outside of the home.

See also – Alienation; Autonomy; Industrialisation

References and further reading

Durkheim, É. (1893/1984) *The Division of Labour in Society*. London: Macmillan.
Smith, A. (1776/1991) *The Wealth of Nations*. London: Everyman's Library.

Early experiences

The term 'early experiences' is typically applied to children under five years of age (in early childhood) as this is often seen as a key developmental period in psychological literature. There is, in fact, a vast research literature on the developmental importance of an individual's early years. The basic assumption is that a person's early relationships and experiences have a profound effect, and ongoing impact, on their cognitive, social and emotional development throughout their life.

The very early years of life are seen as important to children's development as well as for later adult wellbeing. In particular, attachment relationships, parenting style and the material and environmental circumstances of a person's early years have been shown to affect educational attainment in childhood and adolescence as well as emotional wellbeing later in life. Early experiences of poverty, abuse and neglect can have a profound impact on development because of the way a child's natural, innate abilities and vulnerabilities can be negatively influenced and damaged by these external environmental factors.

Government investment in early years services and facilities is a response to this and is seen as beneficial to learning and development because of the way that positive early experiences and support can prevent problems and difficulties developing in later life.

In psychodynamic terms, a person's early childhood experience is seen to play a crucial part in their later development. For example, traumatic and confusing events that have been repressed or pushed into the unconscious are thought to 'leak out' in dreams, irrational behaviour and in psychological distress because the emotional pain linked to them has not been dealt with.

See also – Child abuse; Families; Freud; Psychodynamic perspective; Separation (and loss)

Further reading

Conkbayir, M. and Pascal, C. (2014) *Early Childhood Theories and Contemporary Issues*. London: Bloomsbury.

Dowling, M. (2014) *Young Children's Personal, Social and Emotional Development*, 4th edition. London: SAGE Publications.

Eating disorders

The term eating disorders is used within both mainstream mental health services and popular discourse to describe a group of 'disorders' characterised by unusual eating habits.

The concept of eating disorder is typically based on a severely restricted diet, purging of food from the body or excessive food intake. Eating disorders are typically underpinned by, and are an expression of, mental distress. An eating disorder may lead to acute, long-term or even fatal health consequences for an individual who experiences it.

Eating disorders are associated with western, developed societies where there is no food scarcity. Eating excessively (bingeing) and then vomiting (bulimia) or severely restricting or avoiding consuming food (anorexia) tends to start during adolescence and is much more likely to affect girls and women than boys and men. Eating disorders have been explained in a range of ways, some drawing on biology (brain dysfunction, genetic predisposition) whilst others are rooted in psychological understanding (consequences of abuse, attachment and development issues, identity management and control). Often a person with an eating disorder fears gaining weight, changing body shape and may view their body as too large, repulsive or unusual compared to others. Vomiting, using laxatives and excessive exercise may be used alongside restricted dietary intake to control body weight and development.

A purely biological understanding of eating disorder has limited usefulness. People who experience eating disorders often have coexisting mood disorders (especially anxiety and depression) and may harm themselves. The fact that girls and young women are much more likely to experience an eating disorder than boys and young men has also led to social scientists exploring the issue from feminist standpoints. Gender expectations and stereotypes, the sexualisation of girls and young women in the media and pressure for girls and women to look, act and feel certain ways have been seen as triggers for eating disorders. In this respect, eating disorders are a psychological and political response – a way of asserting and maintaining control in the face of patriarchal pressure.

See also – Mental illness; Patriarchy; Psychiatry

Further reading

Ogden, J. (2010) *The Psychology of Eating: from healthy to disordered behavior*, 2nd edition. Malden, MA: Wiley-Blackwell.

Emotion

Emotion is a state of feeling – a subjective or felt experience of pleasure or displeasure.

There is no scientific agreement on what emotion involves. Any emotion involves a brief, sometimes intense, cognitive experience. However, emotion is also linked to mood, temperament and personality. This makes it harder to define. It is problematic, for example, to say that emotion is a purely 'felt' experience in which the person is not actively thinking. This is because the person is likely to be interpreting events and using mental processes to make sense of their experiences whilst also responding emotionally. So, thinking and mental processes seem to be integral to emotion.

For many psychologists, emotion typically involves a subjective, conscious experience that is characterised by biological/physical reactions (e.g. muscle tension) combined with particular mental states (e.g. fear and apprehension). Sociologists also point out that culture and language are also central to the way we label and give specific emotional experiences and states particular meaning. Neuroscientists have also sought to identify and explain the origins and brain-based processes that produce and express human emotion, suggesting that different emotional experiences are rooted in particular patterns of physiological activity. Emotions are now widely viewed as human responses to significant and meaningful internal and external events, as ways of communicating and relating to others and as triggers to motivate adaptive behaviours that, in evolutionary terms, would have contributed to human survival.

See also – Emotional intelligence; Emotional labour

Further reading

Burton, N. (2015) *Heaven and Hell: the psychology of the emotions*. Oxford: Acheron Press.
Turner, J.H. and Stets, J.E. (2011) *The Sociology of Emotions*. New York: Cambridge University Press.

Emotional intelligence

The concept of emotional intelligence refers to a person's ability to recognise, understand and use their own and other people's emotions appropriately and constructively in the way they think and behave, adapt to different situations and achieve goals.

Two key forms of emotional intelligence have been identified:

- *Ability emotional intelligence* (AI) is the cognitive ability to:
  - identify emotions correctly
  - think accurately when emotions are being expressed
  - understand relationships between emotions and the way they change
  - manage emotions effectively.
- *Trait emotional intelligence* (TI) is a feature of personality that is independent of intelligence. It involves being able to accurately understand and control your own emotional self. Being emotionally expressive, having self-awareness and being optimistic are features of TI.

The concept of emotional intelligence has been used to explain how human beings form and sustain effective relationships with others. A person who is empathetic has AI – they can understand and respond appropriately to the emotions of others, even when under pressure themselves. Both AI and TI are important in enabling an individual to process and use emotional information in the various social environments they encounter.

Possessing emotional intelligence is associated with having better mental health and stronger work performance and having leadership abilities. Daniel Goleman (1996) argued that emotional intelligence contributes more to leadership ability and performance than technical expertise or IQ level, for example. In contrast, critics of the concept of emotional intelligence argue that it is not a valid concept – that is, it doesn't describe or explain a true form of intelligence. Critics tend to argue that its significance is overrated and is not well supported by the research studies that have sought to test the claims made about emotional intelligence.

See also – Cognitive perspective; Emotion; Empathy

Reference

Goleman, D. (1996) *Emotional Intelligence: why it can matter more than IQ*. London: Bloomsbury.

Emotional labour

The sociological concept of emotional labour refers to the work or effort that people put into regulating the way they appear, behave and respond to others.

In the first edition of her influential book published in 1983, Arlie Hochschild first suggested that emotional labour underpins the publicly visible facial and bodily displays that occur in certain workplaces. This type of emotional and presentation management is a feature of nursing and healthcare work, for example. Nurses and other healthcare professionals are often conscious of their non-verbal communication and the way they present themselves to patients, families and other professionals in order to manage emotionally charged or sensitive situations, for example. In doing so, they are engaged in 'emotional labour'.

Hochschild described three emotion regulation strategies that people use as part of 'emotional labour':
- *Cognitive* – these involve efforts to change images, ideas and thoughts with the aim of changing feelings associated with them; for example, using positive images of staff and patients and a 'living well' narrative in information about a dementia service to overcome negative stereotypes of this area of healthcare provision.
- *Bodily* – these involve efforts to change physical symptoms to achieve a desired or preferred emotion; for example, consciously relaxing muscles and taking deep breaths to reduce anxiety or agitation.
- *Expressive* – these involve changing or deliberately using expressive gestures (smiles, frowns, use of their hands) to achieve and convey a particular emotion. Smiling, a brief reassuring touch and making positive eye contact to try to relax somebody is an example of this strategy.

Hochschild (2012) argues that emotional labour is an expected part of work roles (such as nursing) that involve:
- face-to-face or voice-to-voice contact with the public
- situations where the worker (e.g. a nurse) is required to produce an emotional state in another person (e.g. relaxing a patient)
- the employer using strategies such as supervision and appraisal to monitor and control the emotional activities of employees.

Hochschild (2012) argues that these expectations and the level of emotional regulation imposed on employees results in individuals becoming estranged, or alienated, from their real feelings in the workplace.

See also – Alienation; Emotion; Empathy

Reference and further reading

Hochschild, A. (2012) *The Managed Heart: commercialization of human feeling*. Berkeley, CA: University of California Press.

Smith, P. (2011) *The Emotional Labour of Nursing Revisited: can nurses still care?* 2nd edition. Basingstoke: Palgrave Macmillan.

Empathy

Empathy involves a person putting themselves in another person's position to appreciate how they feel or what they think about something.

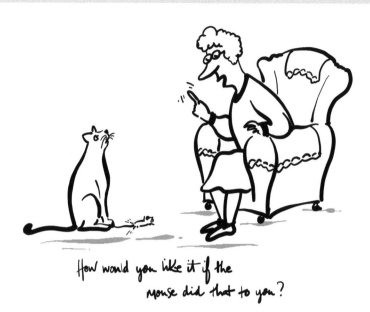

How would you like it if the mouse did that to you?

The concept of empathy originates from humanistic psychology. This has a focus on the self and on developing a holistic understanding that acknowledges and accepts the individual's thoughts, feelings and experiences as being an important part of who they are.

Being empathetic is often quite difficult to do and is distinct from sympathy. The listener needs to put aside any preconceptions they have in order to recognise how the person is struggling to deal with specific problems. They need to be able to 'tune in' to the person's feelings and to use their own emotions intelligently to experience empathy. Empathy does not involve making any guesses or assumptions about what the other person is *really* thinking or feeling. Tschudin (1982) uses the metaphor of helping a man stuck in a ditch to illustrate the difference between empathy and sympathy:

"The sympathetic helper goes and lies in the ditch with him and bewails the situation with him. The unsympathetic helper stands on the bank and shouts 'come on, get yourself out of that ditch!' The empathic helper climbs down to the victim but keeps one foot on the bank and is thus able to help the victim out of trouble onto firm ground again."

Empathy is an important skill that can be used by health and social care workers in many different situations. It is particularly relevant to situations where a person's emotional wellbeing is fragile or a concern. Health and social care workers can make their interactions with service users, family members and colleagues more effective by using empathy appropriately, gaining insight into the needs and experience of service users in an alert, calm way, without having to actually experience it directly. Using empathy also gives health and social care workers a way of communicating with the real person behind the label of service user, relative or colleague.

See also – Attachment; Ethics; Values

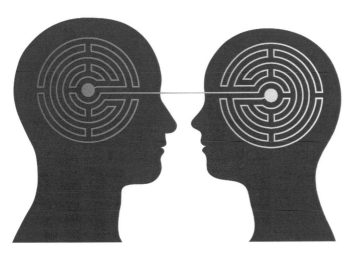

Figure 7 – Empathy involves awareness of another person's feelings and point of view.

Reference and further reading

Baughan, J. and Smith, A. (2013) *Compassion, Caring and Communication: skills for nursing practice*, 2nd edition. Abingdon: Routledge.

Tschudin, V. (1982) *Counselling Skills for Nurses*. London: Bailliere Tindall.

Epidemiology

> Epidemiology is the study and statistical analysis of the patterns, causes and impact of illness, disease (morbidity) and death (mortality) within defined populations.

Epidemiological data is central to public health work as it provides the evidence base for health and social care policy-making, service commissioning and emergency planning and response activities. Epidemiological data on morbidity typically identifies the prevalence rate (the number of people experiencing a condition at a particular time) and the incidence rate (the number of examples of a condition over a particular period such as a year). An epidemiological study may be purely descriptive or can be analytical. A descriptive study simply identifies the who, what, why, how many or how often aspects of a health and illness pattern within a population. An analytical study aims to identify possible causal factors that could explain how and why a disease condition appears within and impacts a population. However, it's important to note that epidemiological studies cannot, by themselves, prove a causal relationship. Specific causation is beyond the realm of epidemiology – it is limited to identifying whether a factor or agent can cause a disease, not whether it has done so.

Epidemiologists use the data they collect to identify risk factors for disease conditions, to explain patterns and variations in rates, incidence and distribution of illnesses and deaths and to shape planning and set targets for preventive healthcare programmes. Epidemiological data also informs evidence-based practice in healthcare. Analysis of the impact of health interventions such as immunisation programmes, health education campaigns or the health promotion strategies used by healthcare workers on health experiences provides useful population-level data that can improve frontline practice, for example.

Epidemiology draws on a wide range of sociological concepts including, for example, gender, ethnicity and consumption patterns when analysing health and illness experiences. Epidemiologists, like sociologists, are interested in population-level patterns rather than individual-level experiences of health and illness. As such, epidemiological studies define their target groups or study populations in an explicit way and make use of sociological concepts and statistical techniques to make causal connections between socio-economic factors (e.g. poverty), patterns of behaviour (e.g. lifestyle, exercise levels) and health outcomes in the group or population being analysed.

See also – Causality; Demography

Further reading

Webb, P., Bain, C. and Page, A. (2015) *Essential Epidemiology: an introduction for students and health professionals*, 3rd edition. Cambridge: Cambridge University Press.

Equalities

In health and social care contexts, equality involves treating everyone who uses care services (or who works within them) in a fair and equal way.

Equality is a wide-ranging term with a number of different meanings. Where people expect to receive equal or fair **access** to treatment or services they are referring to *equality of opportunity* or *equal rights*. The slightly different idea that people are entitled to an equal **share** of health and social care resources (e.g. a practitioner's time or a particular drug treatment) is summed up by the concept of *equity*. Where treatment is provided equitably, every service user will receive their fair share of resources.

The various forms of social inequality that exist in British society can lead some people to experience social exclusion and the negative health effects of social disadvantage, prejudice and unfair discrimination. These effects can be seen in the higher rates of illness, disease and premature death that people in the lower social classes and those in marginalised groups experience. It is important to note that social inequality is not a consequence of the physical, social or cultural differences that exist in the population. It is the unequal distribution of economic and social resources, prejudice and unfair discrimination and the inability, or reluctance, of governments, organisations and individuals to tackle sources of privilege and social advantage that have the effect of creating and maintaining social inequalities.

See also – Advocacy; Discrimination; Diversity; Inequalities

Further reading

Wilkinson, R. and Pickett, K. (2010) *The Spirit Level: why equality is better for everyone.* New York: Bloomsbury.

Ethics

One way of explaining 'ethics' is to see them as principles linked to a fundamental sense of 'right' and 'wrong', 'good' and 'bad'. From this perspective, we all have a set of 'ethics' that guide our behaviour. The ethics we abide by provide us all with a set of moral norms or benchmarks that influence our standards of personal and professional behaviour.

Health and social care practitioners are often faced with sensitive and difficult situations in which they have to make a decision. These could include, for example:

- Should I refer this person for an investigative scan or 'wait and see' whether further symptoms develop?
- Should this person be detained against their will in a mental health unit?
- Is it time to stop giving this person potentially life-saving CPR as they don't seem to be responding or should we carry on in the hope that they will?
- Should we keep this person on a life-support machine or should we switch it off?

In situations like these, there is often no obvious or clearly correct answer. Health and social care practitioners face ethical dilemmas when they have to work out what the 'right' (ethical) course of action is.

As well as providing guidance on how to behave (such as to 'protect confidentiality' or 'accept diversity'), the ethics and care values that health and social care workers draw on point them towards morally acceptable ways of behaving and relating to others. Ethical principles and care values tell us how we *ought* to behave and provide us with benchmarks or norms against which to assess our own and other people's attitudes, decisions and behaviour. They are vital in helping health and social care workers deal with the frequent ethical dilemmas they face.

See also – Equalities; Human rights; Values

Further reading

Chadwick, R. and Gallagher, A. (2016) *Ethics and Nursing Practice*, 2nd edition. London: Palgrave.

Cuthbert, S. and Quallington, J. (2017) *Values and Ethics for Care Practice*. Banbury: Lantern Publishing.

Gallagher, A. and Hodge, S. (2012) *Ethics, Law and Professional Issues: a practice-based approach for health professionals*. Basingstoke: Palgrave Macmillan.

Ethnicity

Social scientists distinguish between 'race' and ethnicity. The concept of 'race' refers to characteristics that are biologically based, such as skin colour. Ethnicity is a broader concept that refers to a social group with a shared, distinct cultural identity.

Social scientists often place the term 'race' in speech marks to indicate that they question, and often reject it as an objective or scientific term capable of categorising naturally occurring groups of people. Instead they argue that 'race' is a socially constructed distinction that reflects eighteenth- and nineteenth-century colonialist assumptions about differences between white and non-white people. In fact, 'race' is seen as a consequence of historically powerful value judgements about the 'natural' superiority of 'white' people in comparison to other 'races'.

Social scientists identify social and cultural factors rather than biological characteristics as being more significant when categorising people using the concept of ethnicity. This is a sense of identity based on shared cultural factors that can, but don't have to, have a 'racial' dimension. Using this approach, an ethnic group is a culturally distinct section of the population. Distinctions between ethnic groups can be made by focusing on language, religion, 'race', ancestral homeland or former citizenship, cultural traditions or way of life, for example.

The perception of cultural 'difference' from others and a felt sense of belonging to a subset of people is made by members of an ethnic group. For example, people who have a common former citizenship, such as Syrians, West Indians or Ethiopians, can be seen to constitute specific ethnic groups in Britain. Alternatively, an 'ethnic group' may be seen to consist of a sub-societal group that has a common descent and cultural background. For example, Romany gypsies and British 'Italian' people are seen to be ethnically distinct for this reason. Finally, an 'ethnic group' can consist of pan-cultural groups with widely differing cultural and social backgrounds who share a similar language, race or religion. 'Asians' are an example of the way this category is used in Britain. People may be identified as 'Asian' despite their apparently different religious affiliations (Hindu, Muslim, Sikh, for example), ancestral homelands (Bangladesh, Pakistan, India), and their diverse languages (Hindi, Punjabi, Bengali) and cultural traditions.

See also – Culture; Identity; Identity politics; Intersectionality

Further reading

Holland, K. and Hogg, C. (2010) *Cultural Awareness in Nursing and Healthcare: an introductory text*, 2nd edition. London: Hodder Arnold.

Evaluation

In the social sciences, evaluation is part of an assessment process. It involves making a judgement about the amount, number, or value of something and is usually the focus of a research investigation or cost–benefit analysis.

Evaluations in the health and social care field tend to make use of measurement devices such as 'performance indicators', attitude surveys, audits or focus groups where qualitative rather than quantitative data is obtained. Evaluations are usually focused on assessing whether specific objectives have been achieved or whether planned interventions have been effective. An evaluation may be formative (assessing progress or impact before a process, change or intervention has been fully completed) or summative (assessing outcomes on completion). The objectives of an evaluation are usually defined by the stakeholder funding the research or analysis project. Data/information or feedback that informs an evaluation should be obtained from parties affected by the intervention, policy or change being evaluated. This may include practitioners, service users, families, service managers and other agencies or organisations affected by the activities being evaluated.

See also – Data; Research methods

Further reading

Ellis, P. (2016) *Understanding Research for Nursing Students*, 3rd edition. London: Learning Matters.

Lindsay, B. (2007) *Understanding Research and Evidence-Based Practice*. Exeter: Reflect Press.

Families

The family is a micro-sociological concept that refers to a primary group of people connected by kinship, marriage or other very close ties, that includes two or more generations. Families also form socio-economic units where the care of children takes place.

Social scientists find defining 'the family' fraught with difficulty. It is generally accepted that there is no such thing as 'the family' in the sense that a wide variety of family forms exist in contemporary society. There is no ideal type or universal version of 'the family'. Examples of family types identified by sociologists include:

- Nuclear family
- Extended family
- Blended/step-family
- Lone parent family
- Domestic partnerships
- Family of choice.

A variety of reasons have been put forward to account for the fact that family diversity is a feature of contemporary society. These include, for example, large scale migration between societies, mobility within societies for work, education or other social reasons, the influence of feminism, shifting class structures, changes in attitudes towards sex, gender and sexuality, changing patterns of marriage, divorce and cohabitation as well as general shifts in social and cultural attitudes and the development of legislation that promotes human rights and equality more broadly.

Sociological accounts of the family have focused on the role it services, as a social institution, for society in general. From a functionalist perspective, the family has been seen to serve several functions, including reproduction, childcare and protection, management of sexual relations, and as a primary economic unit supporting its members. From more critical, conflict perspectives the family has also been seen as playing a key role in preparing and maintaining its members for the workforce, thereby sustaining and fulfilling the labour needs of capitalism.

Sociologists often dispute popular and media portrayals of a past 'golden age' of harmonious family life in which family relationships were a source of social stability, mutual support and nurturing for family members. There has been no such historical period. Nostalgic ideas about the family tend to be based on inaccurate and unrealistic claims that ignore evidence of higher death rates, child abuse and poverty, family breakdown and unstable marriages in periods such as the Victorian era. The presentation of the family as a unit that nurtures and protects its members is questioned by sociologists such as Pahl (1989) who suggests that it's also important to acknowledge that families are often based on unequal power relations that benefit some members but not others. Similarly, social scientists using feminist perspectives have produced a lot of work on the way in which it has become associated with a gendered, private, domestic sphere that relies on women's unpaid labour and restricts their opportunities in the external public sphere of the workplace. Despite questioning the gendered basis of housework and childcare as long ago as the 1970s, women's lives remain much more closely linked to managing, maintaining and reproducing 'family life' than men's. Feminist research and writing has also shone a light on the so-called 'dark side' of family life such as domestic violence, marital rape and the sexual abuse of children that has been neglected in nostalgic and overly positive views of the family as a pillar of society.

See also – Emotional labour; Patriarchy; Social action and social structure; Violence (and aggression)

Reference and further reading

Pahl, J. (1989) *Money and Marriage*. London: Palgrave.

Family therapy

Family therapy involves a range of techniques and strategies that aim to help families deal with relationship problems and to function more effectively and harmoniously. It is a particular type of group therapy and is unusual in UK health and social care settings where individual (one-to-one) and group therapies delivered to groups of unrelated individuals are far more common.

A number of different types, or forms, of family therapy exist. Most are based on the idea that rigid rules and repeating patterns of behaviour within a family can be destructive. For example, blaming, scapegoating, shouting at, physical abuse or the isolation or withdrawal of particular family members may be a feature of a poorly functioning family. These types of negative behaviour may be seen by the family therapist as a way in which the family 'solves' the internal difficulties they have but are ultimately destructive to the individuals who experience them and to the family as a whole.

The systems approach to family therapy is widely used and is an influential way of understanding and addressing problems within families. It suggests that family relations and the behaviours of individuals within the family are part of a 'system'. The implications of this are that the way each person behaves affects the behaviour of others. Consequently, because all behaviours are linked within a family, the pattern of behaviour and relationships must be considered as a whole.

Simply identifying and trying to treat the 'problem behaviours' of one or two individuals will not solve broader family dysfunction. The role of the family therapist is to offer an 'outside view' of what is going on within a family, from a neutral, outsider position. Whilst this can be helpful, taking a neutral, non-judgemental approach to some forms of destructive behaviour is seen as inadequate by critics of family therapy.

In practice, a family therapist may well suggest new ways in which family members could behave, communicate with and respond to each other in order to create or introduce a more positive communication system and family environment. Ultimately, family members – and the family as a group – are responsible for making the changes that are needed for them to relate and live more harmoniously. The family therapist can promote a change in attitudes, viewpoints and behaviours within a family system but can never make this happen without cooperation and effort on the part of family members.

See also – Group therapy; Psychological interventions; Social learning theory

Further reading

Dallos, R. and Draper, R. (2015) *An Introduction to Family Therapy: systemic theory and practice*, 3rd edition. Maidenhead: Open University Press.

Feminism

Feminism is a critical sociological perspective that focuses on women's experiences in society. It is particularly concerned with the inequalities, forms of oppression and unfair discrimination that women experience because of their gender. Feminism has played an important part in the way sociologists think about society since the 1960s.

Feminists criticised both the functionalist and Marxist perspectives in sociology for ignoring the specific experiences and concerns of women. The feminist perspective has been widely applied to areas such as the family, health and care, the education system and employment to highlight inequalities in the opportunities and experiences of men and women and to campaign for change. Marxist, radical and liberal feminism are the three main forms of feminism used in contemporary sociology.

Marxist feminism

Marxist feminists use the conflict model of Marxism to explain how women are exploited, both in terms of social class and gender, in a male dominated society. Women are oppressed and exploited, especially through unpaid domestic and childcare work, by men. They are expected to meet the needs of men, looking after and supporting them, so that men can go out to work. Women are given the primary responsibility of caring for children and ensuring that the home is comfortable and clean. The 'culture of domesticity' and the housewife/mother role that is imposed on women are part of a false consciousness that restricts women's lives and limits their social, educational and employment opportunities. The Marxist feminist perspective offers a structural, conflict viewpoint of society that prioritises the experiences of women.

Radical feminism

Radical feminists view society in terms of a basic and profound conflict of interests between men and women. Society is seen as **patriarchal** and organised in a way that ensures men have power and remain in a dominant position in relation to women. Radical feminists question many of the taken-for-granted female social roles (such as housewife/mother) and attitudes towards women, believing them to be a form of oppression. The answer to this for some radical feminists, is for women to avoid contact with men and to live separate lives. Some radical feminists did set up separatist women-only communities in the 1970s and 1980s that excluded men and which tried to avoid patriarchal forms of social organisation, such as 'family' structures. Radical feminism highlighted the way in which gender equality issues, including domestic violence and sexual assault, were a consequence of repressive male power. This was very influential in the creation of women's centres, rape crisis and domestic violence services and the idea that 'sisterhood' is a powerful way to challenge patriarchy.

Liberal feminism

Liberal feminists adopt a reforming rather than a radical approach to women's experiences and opportunities within society. Liberal feminists are particularly concerned with achieving equality of opportunity in the society that we have, rather than in overturning the current social system. The liberal feminist perspective has been used to identify and explore how sexual discrimination acts as a major barrier to women's equality, for example. The liberal feminist perspective questions the 'naturalness' of gender-specific roles (such as the domesticated housewife/mother and breadwinning husband/father) by pointing out that they are the result of social expectations and processes rather than biological differences between men and women. The liberal feminist perspective has also been used to challenge and change many examples of social disadvantage and gender discrimination, to develop laws on sex discrimination and equal pay and to challenge sexist ideas about women's roles, relationships and place in society.

Weaknesses and criticisms of feminism

Table 6 identifies a number of specific criticisms of Marxist, radical and liberal feminism. In general, feminism has made a positive, constructive contribution to the sociological study of health and social care. It has drawn attention to the different needs and experiences of women as a group and the importance of gender as a social difference that makes a difference to people's lives.

Table 6 – Criticisms of the various types of feminist perspectives

Feminist perspective	Weaknesses and criticisms
Marxist feminism	• Marxist feminists focus too much on class and ignore the powerful influence of other social factors, such as ethnicity, age and disability, on women's lives • Some feminists reject the idea that gender inequalities are caused by capitalism (as opposed to patriarchy or unequal laws)
Radical feminism	• Radical feminists have tended to be white, middle-class women who haven't taken the experiences of black or working-class women into account • Radical feminism's solution of separatism and its rejection of men as a whole is seen as extreme and off-putting because it undermines the interests and views of many women
Liberal feminism	• Liberal feminists are criticised for accepting existing social inequalities (based on class and ethnicity) between women • The liberal feminist goal of 'equality of opportunity' does not challenge the basic assumptions and way of organising society (e.g. roles in the family) that disadvantage women

See also – Gender; Marxism; Socialism

Further reading

Adichie, C.N. (2014) *We Should All be Feminists*. London: Fourth Estate.

Freud

Sigmund Freud (1856–1939) was an Austrian doctor who developed the theory and clinical practice of psychoanalysis.

Freud first qualified as a medical practitioner, a physician, but gradually developed an interest in neurology. This led to him setting up a private medical practice for the treatment of nervous diseases in Vienna in 1886. Freud learnt a lot about human psychological development, particularly psychopathology, from the patients he treated. Freud was particularly interested in the connections between abnormal behaviour and unconscious, underlying psychological processes. He would sit and listen as his, mainly female, patients talked about their anxieties and fears. He also developed and used techniques such as free association, dream analysis and hypnosis to bring unconscious, unresolved conflicts into conscious awareness. Freud believed he could use these techniques to release a person's unconscious conflicts and thereby enable them to deal with their repressed thoughts and feelings. Overall, Freud's psychoanalytical therapy aimed to give the individual in therapy a deep insight into their psyche and personality and greater control and understanding over their emotional life.

Freud learnt a lot about human psychological development, particularly psychopathology, this way. His therapy sessions would often focus on the childhood memories and traumas experienced by his patients. Freud's ideas about the importance of early experiences and the human psychosexual development emerged out of this psychoanalytic practice.

Early psychosexual development

Freud believed that human beings go through several stages of psychosexual development and that early experiences play an important part in this. During this process a child's libido (energy) is focused on the part of their body relevant to that stage.

If the needs of a developing child are met at a particular stage, they can move on to the next stage. If the child struggles or experiences conflict at a particular stage of their development, they may become 'fixated'. Freud argued that this could result in their personality being shaped in a particular way.

Table 7 – Freud's stages of psychosexual development

Stage of development	Focus	Reasons for, and effects of 'fixation'
Oral (0–18 months)	Mouth (sucking, licking, biting)	• Child weaned too early – may develop pessimistic, sarcastic personality • Child weaned too late – may develop gullible, naively trusting personality
Anal (1–3 years)	Toilet training	• Child pressurised to begin toilet training or caught in battle of wills about it may retain faeces to deny parents control and satisfaction – may lead to obstinate, miserly or obsessive personality • Lack of toilet training boundaries – may lead to messy, creative and disorganised personality

Table 7 – Continued

Stage of development	Focus	Reasons for, and effects of 'fixation'
Phallic (3–6 years)	Sex and gender	• Child may be filled with anxiety and guilt about unconscious rivalry with same-sex parent for affection of opposite-sex parent • Boys experience 'castration anxiety', girls experience 'penis envy' • If not resolved may become homosexual/lesbian which Freud believed 'abnormal'
Latency stage (6 years to puberty)	Social pursuits e.g. friendships, sport, academic achievement	• Not strictly a psychosexual development stage • Focus is on social development
Genital stage (puberty to maturity)	Sexual relationships	• More easily negotiated if no previous fixations • If earlier conflicts resolved, will have ability to form warm, loving heterosexual relationship

The Id, the Ego and the Super-ego

Freud's interest in unconscious mental processes also led him to outline a theory about the structure and dynamics of the mind. Freud claimed that the development and expression of a person's emotions and behaviour are driven by three interrelated mental structures – the Id, Ego and Super-ego. According to Freud, the Id and Super-ego are always in conflict. The Id, or unconscious part of the personality, is focused on getting what it wants. It consists of sexual, aggressive and loving instincts and wants immediate gratification. The Super-ego is the last part of the personality to develop as a result of socialisation. Morals and a sense of right and wrong drive it – it is the person's 'conscience'. The Ego tries to balance the demands of the Id and Super-ego. It is the conscious, rational part of the personality.

Freud believed that these three structures or territories of the human mind all affect the way we function psychologically. However, we are not always aware of the actions of, or the interactions between them. A person's conscious mind (Ego) is aware of the here and now. It functions when a person is awake so that the individual behaves in a rational, thoughtful way. The conscious mind handles all the information a person receives from the outside world through their senses. The preconscious mind lies just below the surface of consciousness and contains partially forgotten ideas and feelings. It can be compared to a filing cabinet where we store everything we need to remember and which we can easily bring to conscious awareness. It also prevents disturbing unconscious memories from surfacing. The unconscious mind (Id) is the biggest part and acts as a store of all the memories, feelings and ideas that the individual experiences throughout life. The things that lurk deep in the unconscious are seen within psychodynamic theory to play a powerful, ongoing role in influencing a person's emotions, behaviour and personality.

Sigmund Freud's contribution to psychology is now extremely well known. Many of his ideas, such as the unconscious, the Ego and 'Freudian slips' have entered popular culture and everyday language. However, Freud's contribution to and influence on contemporary mental health practice is marginal. Outside of the very specialist world of psychoanalysis, few mainstream mental health practitioners currently draw on his ideas or use the clinical techniques associated with psychoanalysis.

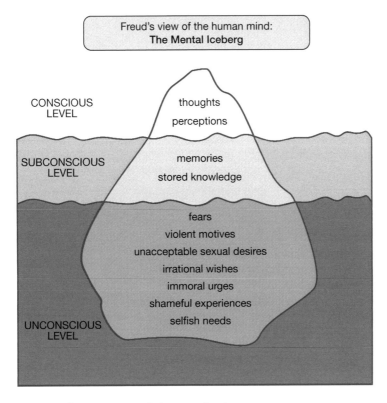

Figure 8 – Freud's view of the human mind: the mental iceberg.

See also – Defence mechanisms; Early experiences; Psychoanalysis; Psychodynamic perspective; Unconscious mind

Further reading

Snowden, R. (2017) *Freud: the key ideas*. London: Teach Yourself.
Storr, A. (2001) *Freud: a very short introduction*. Oxford: Oxford University Press.

Functionalism

Functionalism is a sociological perspective that explains society in terms of inter-linked social structures that perform important roles for society as a whole. Functionalism, like Marxism, is a sociological perspective that sees society as being made up of interconnected parts.

The functionalist perspective is based on the idea that societies are complete systems and that the parts within them cannot be understood in isolation from each other. The functionalist perspective uses a biological metaphor to describe this. Just as the heart, lungs and brain work together to maintain human life, so the family, education system and the law (for example) work together to maintain society. Where the human body consists of interdependent organs, society consists of interdependent social institutions. Each social institution has a particular function or contribution to make to society as a whole. Each social institution must also function effectively and link with others appropriately in order for society to work as it should. Functionalists typically refer to society as a 'social system' to express this idea of an interlinked, interdependent network of social institutions.

Functionalists believe that the structure of society is designed to achieve harmony and agreement between people. Marxists, on the other hand, opt for a conflict view. This highlights social differences and the conflicting interests and values of different groups in society.

Functionalism and the family

Talcott Parsons (1902–1979) was an American sociologist who developed important aspects of the functionalist perspective in the mid-twentieth century. He believed that social institutions, such as the family, had the role of socialising people to behave in acceptable ways so that order was maintained in society. Functionalists see the family as a key social institution in society. G.P. Murdock (1949) produced a classic functionalist study of the family in which he claimed that every known society, from large, developed societies to small hunter-gatherer tribal societies, contained some form of 'family' institution. Murdock identified four key functions of the family in each of these societies:

1. A sexual function, where the family is seen as the approved context or site for the expression of sexual behaviour
2. A reproductive function, where the family is seen as the best, most stable site or context for producing and rearing children
3. A socialisation function, where the family is given the main responsibility for teaching children how to behave in society
4. An economic function, where the family is given the responsibility for providing its members with food, shelter and financial security.

Parsons (1951) also saw the family as pivotal in society, arguing that its basic functions were:
- the primary socialisation of children
- stabilisation of adult personalities (looking after and nurturing adults, especially the male breadwinner).

Critics of functionalism argue that it has a number of weaknesses. In particular, they argue that functionalism:
- ignores conflict and competition in society and paints an overly positive picture of the shared goals and values underpinning society
- focuses on the positive social functions of social institutions and roles and ignores any negative or harmful consequences; for example, adoption of the sick role by people with chronic problems and disability discourages full participation in society and may lead to dependency

- is based on notions of value consensus and assumes this underpins socialisation; however, in a diverse society many different, competing and at times antagonistic value systems coexist.

See also – Interactionism; Marxism; Social action and social structure; Sociological perspective

References and further reading

Dillon, M. (2014) *Introduction to Sociological Theory: theorists, concepts and their applicability to the twenty-first century*, 2nd edition. Chichester: Wiley-Blackwell.

Murdock, G.P. (1949) *Social Structure*. New York: Macmillan.

Parsons, T. (1951) *The Social System*. New York: Free Press.

A
B
C
D
E
F
G
H
I
J
K
L
M
N
O
P
Q
R
S
T
U
V
W
X
Y
Z

Gender

> 'Gender' refers to the cultural and social attributes or expectations of men and women in society that are learnt through socialisation and expressed through notions of masculinity and femininity.

Sociologists make a distinction between the terms 'sex' and 'gender'. 'Sex' tends to be used to refer to the specific, but limited, biological differences between men and women. As such, social scientists argue that discussions, and subsequent understanding, of women's health issues, should be located in the context of gender relations and women's ongoing struggle against gender inequality. So, 'being a woman' isn't just about being biologically 'female' in simple sex terms. It is also about living within a social environment where gender relations, expressed for example through discourses of 'femininity' and 'masculinity', have a profound effect on women and men's social status, their roles and responsibilities and on their different access to power and material resources.

The traditional binary division of male/masculine and female/feminine genders has become a focus of social and political debate in recent years. Specifically, the naturalness and apparent permanence of gender roles associated with men and women has been challenged by those who do not experience their gender in the traditional male or female way or who have sought to switch gender and have transitioned from male/masculine to female/feminine gender status.

Sociologists argue that, because social experience is 'gendered' in various ways, there are significant gender divisions in contemporary society. Differences in the experience of health and illness, and in patterns of mortality, are forms of gender division that are relevant for nurses and other healthcare workers.

Gender and patterns of health and illness

Mortality rates for both sexes have been declining since the mid-nineteenth century. More recently, since 1971, death rates have decreased by 29% for males and by 25% for females, although women continue to have a longer life expectancy than men. Causes of death vary too, with males more likely to die from cancer and heart disease. The pattern of mortality also varies; the age-specific mortality rates for males are higher throughout life, but peak between 15 and 22, with the higher rates of death as a result of motor vehicle accidents. In childhood, boys are far more likely to die from accidents than are girls.

However, the differences are not so clear when it comes to morbidity. Overall, once age is taken into account, there is little difference in the proportions of males and females reporting limiting long-standing illnesses (women live longer and are therefore more likely to report ill health in their final years). During the child-bearing years of women's lives, they report significantly higher levels of illness. More than two-thirds of people with disabilities in Britain are women – although this is also likely to be partly due to the fact that women live longer than men and are therefore more likely to have disabilities.

See also – Feminism; Intersectionality

Further reading

Connell, R.W. and Pearse, R. (2014) *Gender: in world perspective*, 3rd edition. Cambridge: Polity Press.

Genetics

> Genetics is the scientific study of genes, heredity and genetic variation in living organisms.

Gregor Mendel (1822–1884), a nineteenth-century priest and scientist, is seen as the originator of the modern science of genetics. The experiments he carried out on pea plants established many of the rules of heredity, which are now known as the laws of Mendelian inheritance.

Mendel's big discovery was that biological traits are handed down from parents to their offspring through what he called 'units of inheritance' and which are now known as genes. He also showed that the 'dominant' or 'recessive' nature of these genes determined whether they would be expressed in the new organism.

Modern genetic science has developed beyond studying basic gene function and behaviour but does still include this as a significant focus. The structure, function and distribution of genes and their influence on various diseases, developmental processes and human behaviour is now a major part of modern genetics.

See also – Science

Further reading

Carey, N. (2012) *The Epigenetics Revolution: how modern biology is rewriting our understanding of genetics, disease and inheritance.* London: Icon Books.
Skirton, H. and Patch, C. (2009) *Genetics for the Health Sciences.* Banbury: Scion Publishing.
Vipond, K. (2013) *Genetics: a guide for students and practitioners of nursing and health care,* revised edition. Banbury: Lantern.

Globalisation

Globalisation refers to a range of processes that have the effect of bringing dispersed populations of people into closer contact, creating a single, integrated community of interest or interdependent global society.

Globalisation is a contemporary issue in many areas of social science including sociology, social policy, politics and economics. It is an issue that raises a great deal of debate in the everyday world outside of academia as well as within it. From an academic perspective, Marx's ideas about the likely growth of capitalism and Durkheim's arguments about the spread of the division of labour across societies can be seen as early indicators that social scientists were aware in the nineteenth century of globalising processes. It wasn't until the latter part of the twentieth century that the so-called globalisation thesis became a major issue and area of debate within social science. This thesis suggests that globalisation processes accelerated in the 1970s due to the:

- emergence and power of multinational corporations
- declining power of nation states
- creation of regional economic and political entities like the European Union, the World Bank and the World Trade Organization
- growth of cheap travel and international tourism.

Since this period, mass migration of economic migrants and asylum-seeking refugees, the emergence of the internet, social media and instant digital communication as well as the growth of supranational trading blocs has, in many ways, made the world a much smaller place and reshaped societies and global social relations.

The extent to which globalisation is leading to a single global society is disputed within, and outside of, social science. Social scientists generally recognise that globalising processes are affecting all societies and social relations within them as well as the natural environment (air pollution, global warming, infectious disease spread). They debate and disagree about the underlying causes of these processes. Is it fundamentally an economic or financial process, a political process or one being driven by cultural change? Social scientists point to multidirectional global flows and exchanges of financial, political and cultural products to support their arguments. There is evidence to support each of these approaches so it is reasonable to see globalisation as multifaceted and intensifying.

Some see improvements in global literacy, life expectancy and the trend towards democracy, as well as technological advances, as evidence of the benefits of globalisation. Despite this, there is also considerable popular resistance to globalisation – especially the activities of transnational corporations and bodies such as the European Union – as well as a growth in protests by social movements concerned with rising inequalities, unequal life chances and global environmental change.

See also – Capitalism; Division of labour

Further reading

Deaton, A. (2015) *The Great Escape: health, wealth and the origins of inequality*. Princeton, NJ: Princeton University Press.

Steger, M. (2017) *Globalization: a very short introduction*. Oxford: Oxford University Press.

Group(s)/group dynamics

Social scientists tend to see and define 'groups' as *social* groups, emphasising and exploring various aspects of the social nature of groups. In basic terms, a group is formed when two or more people interact for a specific purpose. The concept of group dynamics focuses attention on the nature and pattern of the interactions that occur between members of a social group or between one group of people and another.

Social groups tend to consist of people who have one or more shared characteristics, are interdependent and have a sense of unity. This is known as the social cohesion approach to groups. However, the idea that groups involve interdependence between members isn't shared by all social scientists. Some social scientists argue that groups consist of people who identify themselves as members of a group – regardless of whether they have shared characteristics, interests or objectives. The social identity approach to groups sees belonging as the more important factor in group development and maintenance.

There are many different types of social group in contemporary society – families, work-based groups, social groups, peer groups, communities and even society as a whole can all be seen as social groups. A sense of social cohesion between group members distinguishes those who belong to and identify with the group from those who don't. A queue of people or the collection of people who catch a bus or train at the same time lack such a sense of social cohesion – they are a collection of individuals rather than a group. By contrast, the members of a social group are likely to have characteristics in common (interests, values, kinship ties), a shared goal or purpose and a wish to interact with each other in some way. As a result, social roles (e.g. leader, follower), status ranks and group norms (ways of behaving) are likely to develop in social groups. Acknowledging that social groups are structured and function according to rules and patterns of interaction has led social scientists to explore group dynamics.

The concept of group dynamics refers to the patterns of behaviour and the psychological processes that occur within a social group. In this context, social groups are often seen as behaviour and interaction systems. As such, it is through the relationship dynamics of a social group that group norms, roles, goals and relationships emerge, develop and are maintained. The particular way in which group dynamics operate in a social group has a profound effect on the character of the group. Political, faith-based, military, sports and social groups are likely to operate in different ways and have different characters because they are organised and operate differently. However, the interdependence of group members, the collective 'conscience' of the group, the informal rules that affect behaviour and relationships within the group and between group members and outsiders are all features that are common to social groups. Additionally, social groups may contain internal subgroups and boundaries that affect the dynamics and relationships that exist within the group.

Group dynamics are often an issue in mental health settings where group therapy occurs. Similarly, families are often seen as social systems by many health and social practitioners. An understanding of group dynamics can help practitioners to understand behaviour and relationships in the family as well as plan and deliver interventions aimed at improving communication, cohesion or interaction between family members. Health and social care workers who work as part of a broader healthcare team may also develop an understanding of group dynamics through their own experiences of in-group processes and interactions. This can also be the explicit focus of individual and group supervision sessions where team members are encouraged and supported to discuss and explore the way that group dynamics are impacting on the functioning and effectiveness of the team.

See also – Group therapy

Further reading

Berne, E. (2016) *Games People Play: the psychology of human relationships*. Harmondsworth: Penguin Life.

Cole, M.B. (2017) *Group Dynamics in Occupational Therapy: the theoretical basis and practice application of group intervention*, 5th edition. Thorofare, NJ: SLACK, Inc.

Group therapy

Group therapy is a type of psychotherapy that involves a therapist (or a team of therapists) working with several people (a group) who have similar problems or shared interests. In addition to the psychological interventions that occur within the group, the communication, social interactions and relationship dynamics between group members and the group leaders play an important part in the therapeutic process.

Group therapy generally involves six to ten people meeting regularly with one or two group therapists. There can be a variety of different reasons and purposes for meeting. Groups can be used to deliver different forms of psychological therapy, including cognitive behavioural, interpersonal and psychodynamic therapies. However, the term 'group therapy' is generally associated with forms of group psychotherapy that are based on psychodynamic/psychoanalytic theories and techniques.

A general assumption of group psychotherapy is that the interactions between people in the group will replicate the problems that brought them to group therapy in the first place. As a result, the processes and dynamics of the group can be used to illustrate and understand these problems and are also a mechanism for changing the attitudes, feelings and behaviour of group members. In some cases, group therapy has a purely supportive purpose. It is used to give people who have had similar (often negative or difficult) experiences opportunities to share these experiences with others who are likely to be understanding and supportive. Alternatively, a group may be used to find out about and try out different, more positive ways of relating to other people. For example, a person may share their feelings of low self-esteem and lack of confidence but go on to test out different ways of being assertive within the group.

The role of the group therapist is to analyse and monitor the dynamics of the group, facilitate communication and enable members to participate in a safe, supported and productive way. Groups usually negotiate rules relating to confidentiality, boundaries and ways of working that the therapist and group members must always adhere to.

Group therapy is a common feature of both statutory and voluntary mental health and social care settings and is also now often available in private counselling and psychotherapy settings. In addition to 'talking therapy' groups, group therapy may be delivered through dance, drama/psychodrama, music and art therapy groups. Specialist therapeutic community settings, where people live together as a group, also make explicit use of group therapy approaches. In these settings the total environment or milieu of the setting is used as the therapy medium. All workers and members of the therapeutic community are part of the group. Their daily activities and interactions are the focus of regular analysis and discussion, often at a weekly 'community meeting'. Group members can use these meetings to raise issues, make comments about what has been happening or criticise how they have been treated or even be confronted about their attitudes and behaviour towards others.

See also – Cognitive behavioural therapy; Family therapy; Mental illness

Further reading

Bion, W.R. (1998) *Experiences in Groups*. Abingdon: Routledge.
Yalom, I.D. and Leszcz, M. (2005) *The Theory and Practice of Group Psychotherapy*, 5th edition. New York: Basic Books.

Health

Health is a contested concept in the broad medical and health and social care field. It is used in various ways to refer to the functional state of the human body and to the extent to which an individual is free from disease, illness and injury and able to experience a sense of physical, psychological and emotional wellbeing. Definitions of health can be categorised as holistic, negative and positive.

Holistic definitions

The holistic approach to health suggests we should take all aspects of a person's life into account when we're looking at their health. This approach is concerned with the 'whole person' and includes an individual's:
- physical (bodily) health and wellbeing
- intellectual (thinking and learning) wellbeing
- social (relationship) wellbeing
- emotional (feelings) wellbeing.

Many holistic definitions also see spiritual wellbeing as integral to an individual's 'health'.

The term 'wellbeing' is linked to, but can also be differentiated from, health. Wellbeing is used in western societies to refer to the way people feel about themselves. If people feel 'good' (positive) about themselves and are happy with life they will have a high level of wellbeing, and vice versa. As individuals, we are the best judges of our personal sense of wellbeing. From a holistic perspective, health cannot be achieved without wellbeing.

Positive definitions

Positive definitions of health focus on the qualities, characteristics and assets that enable a person to flourish and experience holistic wellbeing. Using a positive approach, the World Health Organization (WHO, 1946) has defined health as being "a state of complete physical, mental and social wellbeing, not merely the absence of disease of infirmity".

What the WHO is doing here is actually providing us with *two* definitions, and making it clear that it supports only the positive definition of health as a *state of complete physical, mental and social wellbeing*. The key term here is 'wellbeing', which seems to suggest that the person feels good both mentally and physically, despite the existence of any 'objective' mental or physical infirmities.

The positive definition of 'health' is vague and unclear in 'medical' terms. It seems to suggest that 'health' has as much to do with general quality of life issues as it does with biology. Alternative health and complementary therapy practitioners tend to use this kind of definition as part of their practice more than traditional medical practitioners do.

Negative definitions

Negative definitions of health focus on the absence of diagnosable disease or illness.

The second part of the quote from the WHO suggests that 'health' is the state of *not* having an illness, infirmity or disease. This is a more commonly used and accepted, though not necessarily a 'truer' or better, way of defining 'health' in the UK. Using this definition, we would say that when a person feels unwell they are 'unhealthy', or lack 'health'. In other words, 'health' is defined by the absence of ill health. Within this definition, a distinction is often made between illness and disease. Illness involves a person's own, or 'subjective', definition of their lack of health, of 'not feeling right' or 'feeling unwell'. However, disease is a biological state in which an individual's body is affected by some form of observable physical 'abnormality' or pathology. The simplest way to understand this is to view the body as a machine that may at times malfunction because, for some reason, one or more of the parts stops working. The damage to the machine part is 'disease'.

Currently, most healthcare practice and policy is based on this type of negative definition. Taking the machine metaphor we used earlier, it is the role of the doctor to identify physical faults and repair them. This is achieved through 'curative medicine', based on surgery and the use of pharmaceuticals (drugs) that alleviate biological disorder.

See also – Biomedical model; Social model of health

Reference and further reading

Barry, A-M. and Yuill, C. (2016) *Understanding the Sociology of Health*, 4th edition. London: SAGE Publications.

World Health Organization (1946) *Constitution: basic documents.* Geneva: WHO.

Humanistic perspective

The humanistic perspective is an approach to psychology that focuses attention on the human capacity for making choices and experiencing psychological and emotional growth. It assumes people have free will, are driven towards self-actualisation and have the same basic needs and values regardless of their life circumstances. Humanistic psychologists see human subjective experience of the world as their primary subject matter.

The humanistic perspective became popular in psychology and began to influence health and social care practitioners from the mid-twentieth century onwards. Abraham Maslow (1908–1970) and Carl Rogers (1902–1987), both American psychologists, are now seen as the pioneers of this perspective. The humanistic perspective adopts a holistic approach to human experience. This involves studying the whole person rather than focusing on a specific aspect or part of them. It is concerned with uniquely human issues and experiences such as the self, self-actualisation (achieving your potential) and individuality.

There is now wide acceptance in the health and social care sectors that an individual's needs, identity and values should always be respected. It is good practice not to criticise or make personal judgements about people who are receiving care, for example. Humanistic psychologists argue that we need to try to identify with other individuals – which can be difficult because of social differences – in order to avoid discriminatory practice and to provide services that meet each individual's needs and preferences. In this way the humanistic principle of valuing the personal worth of each individual is being put into practice.

Understanding and using the self

Carl Rogers (1961), one of the pioneers of humanistic psychology, was interested in the development of the self. He focused on the capacity that people have for self-direction and for understanding their own development needs. Rogers noted that an individual's self-concept is strongly influenced by the judgements they make about themselves and by what they believe others think about them. For example, a negative self-concept can develop if a person internalises critical comments that others make about them ('you're hopeless') and then thinks and acts as if this is true. Rogers was also concerned with the importance of self-esteem and the role of the 'ideal self' in the way that we make judgements about ourselves. Humanistic psychologists such as Rogers (1961) claim that a mismatch between the ideal self and actual self can lead to psychological and emotional problems.

Table 8 – Summary of the strengths and weaknesses of the humanistic approach to psychology

Strengths	Weaknesses/limitations
Recognises that the complexity of human emotions and relationships affects the way people develop and behave	Based on relatively vague, unscientific concepts that can't be tested easily
Provides useful concepts for developing supportive and ethical human relationships	Encourages people to focus on self-fulfilment and perfecting themselves – it can be seen as narcissistic
Sees people as capable of resolving their problems in an individual way	Focuses on the individual rather than on the influence of others or their broader social or cultural surroundings

Table 8 – Continued

Strengths	Weaknesses/limitations
The humanistic perspective encouraged psychologists to accept that there is more to human behaviour and psychological experience than observable behaviour	The humanistic focus on the individual and self-fulfilment can be seen as selfish and narcissistic
Humanism is based on a positive view of human nature that emphasises individual responsibility	Critics see the humanistic perspective as assuming an overly optimistic view of the world; it doesn't recognise that some people are unable to achieve self-fulfilment because they face significant social disadvantages, for example
The ideas and concepts of the humanistic perspective are flexible and can be applied widely in health and social care settings	The ideas and theories of the humanistic perspective can't be tested; they are seen as vague and unverifiable by those who want scientific evidence of effectiveness
The humanistic perspective is based on values that are inclusive and supportive of all human beings	The humanistic perspective suggests that everyone is capable of achieving self-actualisation and self-fulfilment; this may only be true of very talented and socially advantaged people
The humanistic perspective is very client-centred and has enabled a large counselling industry to grow and develop	Humanistic psychology ignores the unconscious – it recognises only those thoughts and behaviours that people are aware of

See also – Psychological perspective; Rogers, Carl; Self-actualisation

Reference and further reading

Gross, R. (2015) *Psychology: the science of mind and behaviour*, 7th edition. London: Hodder Education.

Rogers, C. (1961) *On Becoming a Person: a therapist's view of psychotherapy*. Boston, MA: Houghton Mifflin.

Human rights

Human rights refer to principles, usually expressed as legal rights, which identify or establish standards of behaviour that are expected of people in a society and which everyone in a society is entitled to enjoy.

Human rights are often understood to refer to opportunities (e.g. to worship, marry or speak freely), to ways of being treated or to freedoms that every human being has, or should have, whatever their social, cultural or religious background and wherever they live in the world. They can, therefore, be seen as universal entitlements that express and promote egalitarian values. That is, they support the view that by virtue of being human, every person is entitled to be treated, and is expected to behave, according to certain norms or standards. However, human rights are not innate or naturally occurring phenomena. They depend on education, shared values and the rule of law to introduce, protect and impose them. Human rights are often contested and hotly debated because they encapsulate moral ideas and set standards or norms for what is acceptable and expected in a society. Universal entitlement to human rights means that they cannot be taken away unless a society has agreed legal procedures to override them in specific circumstances. For example, a person who commits a violent offence may have their human right to freedom removed because of laws that require people to be imprisoned for such an offence.

In the UK, the Human Rights Act (1998) sets out the human rights of UK citizens in a series of 'Articles'. Each Article deals with a different right. These are all taken from the European Convention on Human Rights and are commonly known as 'the Convention Rights':

- Article 2 Right to life
- Article 3 Freedom from torture and inhuman or degrading treatment
- Article 4 Freedom from slavery and forced labour
- Article 5 Right to liberty and security
- Article 6 Right to a fair trial
- Article 7 No punishment without law
- Article 8 Respect for your private and family life, home and correspondence
- Article 9 Freedom of thought, belief and religion
- Article 10 Freedom of expression
- Article 11 Freedom of assembly and association
- Article 12 Right to marry and start a family
- Article 14 Protection from discrimination in respect of these rights and freedoms

The concept of a 'right' is controversial and continues to be debated. Many of the debates about human rights focus on which rights should be included in the moral and general framework of human rights. Should the right to health (or healthcare) be included? What about the right to education, or the human rights of the unborn child? Political and other interest groups argue vigorously for the inclusion of their issues and position in the human rights framework. Others resist suggesting that human rights should be a more limited concept that ought to set the minimum standards for acceptable human behaviour and the prevention of abuse.

See also – Autonomy; Data; Ethics

Further reading

Grodin, M., Tarantola, D., Annas, G.J. and Gruskin, S. (eds) (2013) *Health and Human Rights in a Changing World*. Abingdon: Routledge.
Human Rights Act (1998).

Hypothesis

A hypothesis is a provisional claim about something that is not yet supported by evidence.

Social scientists carrying out research investigations based on a scientific approach typically put forward a hypothesis that they then set out to test. Hypotheses typically establish the focus and direction of research studies and are closely linked to what is already known about a phenomenon but which cannot be adequately explained by existing theory or knowledge.

Hypotheses are more likely to be a feature of psychological rather than sociological research studies. This is largely because psychological research is more likely to explore or generate quantitative data, whereas sociologists are more likely to focus on and generate qualitative data in their research studies. Psychological experiments, for example, always begin with a hypothesis which will be tested using scientific methods. The findings of the experiment may result in the hypothesis being proven or remaining unsupported by the evidence. Regardless of the outcome, a hypothesis remains open to further investigation as the variables and/or context in which it is either proven or unsupported may change. Ellis (2016) suggests that a hypothesis has the following key characteristics:

- It suggests the relationship between two or more variables
- It identifies the nature of the relationship
- It points to the research design to be used
- It indicates the population to be studied.

Researchers tend to use their knowledge and experience of an issue, subject or area of practice to generate a hypothesis.

See also – Data; Evaluation; Research methods

Reference and further reading

Ellis, P. (2016) *Understanding Research for Nursing Students*, 3rd edition. London: Learning Matters.

Lindsay, B. (2007) *Understanding Research and Evidence-Based Practice*. Exeter: Reflect Press.

Ideal type

An ideal type, as used in social science, refers to a perfect or idealised example of a social phenomenon. Ideal types tend to focus on the particular, definitive characteristics of the phenomenon being described, so that the similarities and differences of cases in the real world can be compared to the ideal type.

Max Weber (1904/1949), an early pioneer of sociology, developed and used the concept of ideal types in order to engage with and explain some of the complexity of the social world. Weber was clear that ideal types are not real, in the sense that they don't actually exist in the social world. However, by constructing an ideal type of a particular phenomenon (e.g. a capitalist market, consumer society or gender role) it is possible to engage with what is actually happening in the real world by comparing it to the ideal type. The ideal type offers a reference point from which to observe, analyse and try to understand the social world.

Sociologists tend to use ideal types in the early stages of research. They can be useful for generating research questions and hypotheses about the phenomena being studied. This is particularly helpful when social scientists want to study a new social phenomenon. An ideal type can be constructed to guide subsequent investigation into specific cases or examples of the new phenomena. The fact that ideal types oversimplify aspects of the social world and can't adequately represent aspects of social life other than in a stereotypical way is the major criticism of this concept.

See also – Social action and social structure; Sociological perspective; Sociology

Reference

Weber, M. (1904/1949) 'Objectivity in social science and social policy', in E.A. Shils and H.A. Finch (eds), *The Methodology of the Social Sciences*. New York: New York Free Press.

Identity

A person's identity refers to their unique sense of self. It consists of characteristics that are specific to them as an individual as well as characteristics that connect them to others (especially groups). It is about who they are and their sense of belonging as well as who other people think they are.

According to social scientists, an individual's identity is socially developed rather than naturally occurring. Identity develops and is shaped through interaction with others. A person's sense of themselves as an individual is closely related to the identities of other people in their life. In this way identity is relational – a girl's identity is partly affected by being a 'daughter' to her 'mother' (part of a different person's identity) and the way that this mother–daughter relationship is lived out and experienced, for example. As well as being constructed out of what a person thinks and feels about themselves and how they understand and experience their relationships with others, identity is also affected by the way others respond to and treat us. As such, identity is a multi-layered and complex idea.

Jenkins (2014) describes identity as having three parts or layers:
- an individual, personal layer – primary identification of our gender, ethnicity, capabilities and capacities
- a collective or social layer – this refers to our sense of identification with others (who we feel we belong to), our social and occupational roles and statuses
- an embodied layer – who we are and who others see and relate to us as, is partly embedded in us at a physical, bodily level.

Identity development is continuous and never fixed because all of these parts or layers of an individual's identity are fluid and in a state of flux. Identity is socially made and remade; each of is forever subject to and responding to change. The implication of this is that identities are unstable, can be multiple and indicate that we are always in the process of becoming ourselves. A person can also make choices that alter their identification with others, positioning themselves as being similar to or different from others. This doesn't just work one way though – others can also position us on the basis of identity too. Sociologists such as Goffman (1963) discussed this in his study of stigma where a stigmatised characteristic, such as physical disability, mental illness or learning disability for example, can 'spoil' a person's identity by marking them out as different from others.

See also – Alienation; Ethnicity; Gender

References

Goffman, E. (1963) *Stigma: notes on the management of spoiled identity.* Englewood Cliffs, NJ: Prentice-Hall.
Jenkins, R. (2014) *Social Identity*, 4th edition. Abingdon: Routledge.

Identity politics

The concept of identity politics developed in the late twentieth century to describe the political positions that individuals, communities and cultural groups ascribe to (i.e. identify with) in order to express and support particular interests and perspectives.

Identity politics play an important part in the way a person identifies with social and political organisations. In particular, an individual's identification with organisations and communities that have a political, environmental, social change or minority support focus is a way of articulating personal values and demonstrating an affiliation with oppressed and marginalised groups. Identity politics is also concerned with trying to change the marginalised position of oppressed groups. In this sense it has connections to human rights issues and resistance to political power – particularly the power of a nation's dominant individuals, groups and communities. Feminist groups, minority ethnic groups, lesbian, gay and transgender groups and disability rights groups have all developed and organised through identity politics. The politics of identity – focusing on the issue of who you are and what your rights ought to be – have been a major theme of black freedom, gay liberation, women's liberation and disability rights movements since the 1960s, for example. For some members of these groups, the goal of their identity politics is acceptance by and within the mainstream on an equal basis. However, others seek to develop alternative lifestyles and ways of living that are outside of the institutions and culture of mainstream society that they see as profoundly discriminatory and rejecting.

One of the criticisms and weaknesses of identity politics is that groups who are united by an issue, characteristic or shared goal also tend not to explore the differences that exist among themselves. This can be important because these differences (e.g. in social class or gender) can be sufficient to frustrate the group's aims. The concept of intersectionality helps to shed light on why campaigns based on identity politics can generate a lot of concern and debate but little action or change.

See also – Culture; Human rights; Identity; Ideology; Intersectionality

Further reading

Martín Alcoff, L., Hames-García, M., Mohanty, S.P. and Moya, P.M.L. (eds) (2006) *Identity Politics Reconsidered.* New York: Palgrave Macmillan.

Ideology

An ideology is a set of beliefs or ideas that, when combined, can be used to explain, interpret or guide social, political and economic life and action.

The term ideology is difficult to define in a precise way. It was first used by the French writer Antoine Destutt de Tracy, in his book *Eléments d'Idéologie* (1805), to refer to the need to develop a 'science of ideas' in politics. At the time, it was believed that 'ideologies' could provide objective, truthful and scientific approaches to understanding. However, social scientists now see ideologies as having particular purposes and as being used to promote, support and legitimise the interests of dominant groups in society. This chimes with Karl Marx's argument that an ideology is not a neutral set of ideas but is, in fact, a set of false and misleading beliefs, typically propagated by a ruling elite to oppress and exploit the masses.

Whilst not everybody is as critical of ideology as Marx, it is now generally accepted within social science that ideologies are partial accounts of reality and that they carry and communicate an implicit agenda. Political and religious beliefs are often viewed by social scientists as ideological because they express views about how people *ought* to behave and claim to provide a true or correct account of how the social world really works. Ideological beliefs are at their most powerful when they enter public consciousness and provide an unquestioned (and unquestioning) way of interpreting the world and what is happening within it. The social science response to ideological claims is often to point to the way ideologies are linked to power and power relations and are used to hide or justify the agenda and interests of dominant groups in society. Mass media, including social media, are seen as being important in the dissemination of ideological beliefs. Newspapers, magazines, television and radio programmes and now websites, blogs and tweets are all channels through which ideologies can be communicated to large audiences. Similarly, education, the law and healthcare practice have all been seen as sites of ideological activity in which particular sets of ideas and beliefs dominate and determine how we live, understand and experience everyday life. To some extent this is an important socialising process that promotes social cohesion – ideologies communicate values and beliefs and encourage us to abide by shared rules in society, for example.

The concept of ideology remains relevant within social science, though many social scientists now use the concept of discourse to analyse and draw attention to the links between ideas, the ways they are presented and the agendas of powerful interest groups. With the recent emergence and growing importance of social media as a source of (mis)information in society, the notion that 'news', 'data' and 'comment' about political, social and economic issues is ideologically driven rather than neutral or objective has brought the concept back into use and has highlighted the existence of a continuing battle for ideological dominance in society.

See also – Discourse; Power; Socialism

Further reading

Freeden, M. (2003) *Ideology: a very short introduction*. Oxford: Oxford University Press.
Heywood, A. (2017) *Political Ideologies: an introduction*, 6th edition. London: Palgrave.

Industrialisation

Industrialisation refers to the gradual change in methods of production in a society from traditional, agricultural or agrarian methods to those involving some form of mechanised, factory-based production.

Britain was the first nation in the world to go through the process of becoming industrialised. The Industrial Revolution is thought to have begun at some time in the eighteenth century, and it continued into the twentieth century. Historical evidence shows that, during this period, industrialisation transformed British society and the lives of British people. Social transformation did not happen suddenly, as though one year Britain was a pre-industrial, agricultural society and the next it was 'industrialised'. There was a gradual change in methods of production and the location of people's work that – combined with other important social, political and economic developments – are linked to the development of major health and social welfare problems.

At the beginning of the eighteenth century, Britain was primarily an agricultural country with most people living in rural areas. The population of Britain was only nine million (Jones, 1994), but was about to expand rapidly. The majority of workers and industries operated within a domestic system. This involved people working in their own homes to produce goods, or components of goods, and also to cultivate food on their own farm or piece of land. The advantages of this system were that workers and their families were free to work for themselves at their own pace, work and family life were relatively integrated, and working conditions could be controlled by workers. During the eighteenth century there was a gradual move away from this way of working. The invention of machines led to a revolution in the ways in which goods could be produced – and the speed and scale of the process. Work was gradually relocated into factories that housed the machines. This gradual move from domestic to factory-based systems of production did not occur at the same pace in all areas of industry, and varied across the regions of Britain. There is extensive historical evidence, however, that the general process of industrialisation was well under way by 1800 (Brown, 1991).

The eighteenth and nineteenth centuries saw significant changes in the size, location and lifestyle of the British population. Industrialisation was a very important influence in stimulating this movement. The growth of factories and the availability of work in them attracted people from rural areas and sustained higher densities of people in particular areas. This gradual but major shift in the location of the population, and the growth of towns and cities around them, is known as urbanisation.

See also – Poverty; Urbanisation

References

Brown, R. (1991) *Society and Economy in Modern Britain 1700–1850*. London: Routledge.
Jones, K. (1994) *The Making of Social Policy in Britain 1830–1990*. London: The Athlone Press.

Inequalities

The concept of inequality is widely used in economics and sociology. It refers to the uneven distribution of valued resources (monetary, material or opportunities).

Inequality is a multidimensional concept in that it is used to refer to differences, or disparities, in income, wealth, prestige, power and access to resources, amongst other things. Social scientists typically refer to social inequalities – that is, the uneven and unequal distribution of resources according to socially defined categories (e.g. social class, gender, ethnicity) of people. It is also common to see reference being made to *socio-economic* inequalities, particularly within sociological literature. These inequalities refer to unequal distributions of income and wealth according to social class or some other social categorisation. Social inequalities are not just limited to the unequal distribution of financial resources, however. In addition to financial inequality, status, access to power and social opportunities, rights and privileges as well as access to and use of public services (e.g. health, education and housing) are all unevenly distributed in the UK and many other countries. Despite evidence of widespread inequalities in the UK, many people, as well as governments, believe that contemporary society is largely meritocratic. That is, that resources and opportunities are distributed on merit.

Despite this, there is considerable research and statistical data to show that socio-economic inequalities are linked to gender inequalities, racial inequalities and other forms of unfair treatment of marginalised social groups.

The various forms of social inequality that exist in UK society can lead some people to experience social exclusion and the health effects of social disadvantage, prejudice and unfair discrimination. These effects can be seen in higher rates of illness, disease and premature death that those in the lower social classes and those in marginalised groups experience. It is important to note that social inequalities are not a consequence of the physical, social or cultural differences that exist in the population. It is the unequal distribution of economic and social resources, prejudice and unfair discrimination and the inability, or reluctance, of governments, organisations and individuals to tackle sources of privilege and social advantage that have the effect of creating and maintaining social inequalities.

See also – Child poverty; Equalities; Poverty; Social policy

Further reading

Wilkinson, R. and Pickett, K. (2010) *The Spirit Level: why equality is better for everyone.* New York: Bloomsbury.

Interactionism

This term refers to a range of sociological perspectives that focus on detailed aspects of everyday social behaviour and the ability of social actors (individuals and groups) to influence society themselves. The interactionist perspective focuses on the ways in which individuals make choices and on the meanings of social behaviour. This is a very different approach to the structuralist perspectives of functionalism and Marxism because it assumes that people themselves, rather than big social forces such as 'class' or 'gender', can make a difference to society and how we live our lives within it.

Sociologists who use interactionist perspectives believe that it's better to look at the micro-social behaviours of people and the social processes that occur in care settings (care practices, doctor–patient relationships, labelling processes) rather than at the macro-level structures and social trends that occur at a more distant, societal level. Interactionists look at society through a 'microscope' whereas structuralists look at society through a 'magnifying glass'.

Table 9 – Specific criticisms of the interactionist perspective in sociology

Issue	Criticisms
Focus	Interactionism focuses on detailed aspects of social life and ignores the bigger, structural picture. It doesn't see society as a social system.
Uses of research	Interactionist research tends to be small-scale and produces findings that are specific to the research setting. Findings can't be applied to society as a whole.
What makes society 'tick'	Interactionists don't take account of power in society or consider how wider social forces or historical processes can influence social relationships and individuals' interactions.

See also – Social action and social structure; Sociological perspectives

Further reading

Lipscomb, M. (ed.) (2017) *Social Theory and Nursing*. Abingdon: Routledge.

Intersectionality

This concept refers to the idea that a number of different social inequalities or social divisions intersect and become interwoven in the production of social disadvantage, unfair discrimination and social exclusion. As a result, intersectionality is used to explain the complexity and persistence of social inequalities.

The impact of social class on social relations, life opportunities and the structure of society was the focus of many sociologists for much of the twentieth century. The work of Karl Marx in the nineteenth century on class structures and dynamics within capitalism largely motivated this focus on the power of social class to shape society. Consequently, sociologists paid less attention to other social factors and processes that also influenced social experiences, such as gender, ethnicity and culture, for example. However, by the late twentieth century it was clear that social class alone did not and could not provide a sufficient explanation for social inequalities. At the end of the 1980s social scientists began to explore how social divisions in society (around gender, race/ethnicity, sexual orientation and age, for example) 'cut across' and intersected each other. They were interested in how people's lives and identities were affected at the intersection of class, gender and 'race'/ethnicity, for example.

A lot of the early work and subsequent development of social science in this area resulted from an interest in social and cultural diversity and the growth of identity-driven politics. Intersectionality allowed social class to be connected to other forms of social division and also exposed the weakness of sociological work that was based on overgeneralised notions of 'women', the 'working class' or the 'black community', for example. It was realised that members of these groups may not primarily identify with gender, class or ethnicity, for example. Their social identities may be much more complex and nuanced. The life, opportunities and identity of a young, lesbian white working class woman may be very different from that of an older, heterosexual black working class woman, despite their shared class position. Intersectionality draws attention to the social differences and divisions that affect each of these women and points social scientists towards the way that power relations affect their respective lives. It is the particular ways in which intersecting social categories combine that determine how a person experiences the social world. Social scientists applying the concept of intersectionality are interested in the interplay between social positions rather than in the power of a single factor to determine a person's life experiences and opportunities.

Intersectionality has played an important role in helping social scientists to recognise and explore the impact of social and cultural diversity in society. It has been used to show that the impact of social disadvantage may not be evenly spread or uniformly experienced across a class, gender or ethnic group. However, some critics of this approach also argue that in acknowledging the significance of diverse social identities and experiences, intersectionality takes the focus away from the structured patterns of social inequality and disadvantage. Population-level data continues to show, for example, that a person's social class has a profound impact on life chances and mortality rates.

See also – Ethnicity; Gender; Identity; Social class

Further reading

Berger, M.T. and Guidroz, K. (eds) (2010) *The Intersectional Approach: transforming the academy through race, class and gender.* Chapel Hill, NC: University of North Carolina Press.

May, V.M. (2015) *Pursuing Intersectionality, Unsettling Dominant Imaginaries.* New York: Routledge.

Labelling theory

Labelling involves attaching generalised descriptions (labels) to people as a way of summing them up. Labelling should be avoided in health and social care settings as labels are often stigmatising and negative (e.g. diagnostic labels such as 'depressive') and can become a 'master status' that affects the way a person thinks about themselves and the way others treat them. Labelling may also affect the way care practitioners communicate with service users because some labels (such as 'schizophrenic', for example) can lead to insensitive, negative and less favourable treatment.

Labelling theory developed as part of the interactionist perspective within sociology. When applied to the health and social care field, labelling theory has been used to help care practitioners understand what happens during face-to-face interactions. In particular, interactionism has shown how the labelling of behaviour is a social process that has implications for the way people are treated and identify themselves in health and social care settings. Labelling theory has been used to explain how the medical process of diagnosing health problems is, in fact, often a social process. For example, in the nineteenth century women who exhibited a range of symptoms including crying and laughing for 'no reason' were diagnosed with the disease of 'hysteria'.

Medical practitioners at the time believed 'hysteria' was caused by women trying to do activities, such as going out to work, that were beyond their natural abilities. The cure was rest and a return to domestic activity. However, there was no such disease. Labelling the symptoms as illness was in fact a way of controlling and oppressing women. Health and social care practitioners are now aware that using crude diagnostic labels such as 'hysteric', 'schizophrenic' or 'spastic' stereotypes a person in a negative way and can be discriminatory and unhelpful as a way of describing a person's care needs.

See also – Interactionism; Prejudice; Sociological perspective; Stigma

Further reading

Becker, H.S. (1997) *Outsider: studies in the sociology of deviance.* New York: Free Press.
Goffman, E. (1990) *Stigma: notes on the management of spoiled identity.* London: Penguin.

Learning difficulties (and learning disabilities)

Learning difficulties refer to problems learning in typical or expected ways.

The terms 'learning difficulty' and 'learning disability' have historically been used synonymously. This is no longer the case in the UK and many other countries. Learning difficulties tend to be the result of:

- dyslexia – difficulties in reading and writing words fluently
- dyscalculia – difficulties in understanding and using numbers.

'Learning disability' now tends to indicate that a person has an intellectual impairment that affects their overall ability to function (socially and psychologically) and learn. The contemporary focus on 'learning disability' shifts attention away from a person's IQ or level of intelligence to their general social functioning, ability to acquire new skills and understand information and their ability to live independently. The term 'learning difficulty' is too narrow to describe these relatively wide-ranging issues.

Learning difficulty is now used to focus attention directly and specifically on a problem related to learning, rather than on social or psychological functioning. A person may have a generalised learning difficulty that may or may not be linked to their level of intelligence. For example, a child who has a visual or hearing impairment or a physical disability that restricts their ability to access standard educational facilities and resources may experience learning difficulties in mainstream educational settings and may be identified as having special educational needs. Alternatively, a person may have a specific learning difficulty, such as dyslexia, that has no link to their IQ but which affects their ability to learn.

See also – Cognitive development; Cognitive perspective; Developmental norms

Further reading

Barber, C. (2015) *Caring for People with Learning Disabilities*. Banbury: Lantern Publishing.
Talbot, P., Astbury, G. and Mason, T. (2010) *Key Concepts in Learning Disabilities*. London: SAGE Publications.

Life chances

The concept of life chances is used within social science to describe the opportunities each individual has to improve their quality of life. Originally developed by the German sociologist Max Weber, life chances provides a way of predicting or estimating the likely way a person's life will turn out. Sociologists who use this concept tend to see a close connection between a person's socio-economic status (their social class) and their life chances.

A person's opportunities in life tend to be linked to their access to resources. Having enough food to eat and good quality housing are basic resources, for example. Access to good quality education, health and social care services and employment opportunities are also important social and economic resources. Each of these resources affects an individual's quality of life and ability to not just meet but also satisfy their needs. Max Weber and other subsequent social scientists have argued that in addition to economic factors (income and wealth), a variety of other factors including gender, race/ethnicity, social mobility and equality issues all affect an individual's life chances.

A key debate in this area is whether a person's life chances are determined by factors beyond their control (such as their class, gender and ethnicity) or not. The alternative argument is that individuals do have some influence, or agency, to affect their life chances through their own conduct and decision-making. In particular, people have control over their values and beliefs and have the capacity to make decisions and choices that affect their life at different points. In this sense a person is not helpless or powerless to affect the course of their life. However, if a society offers fewer or poorer quality opportunities to some groups compared to others because it is socially unequal, then those in the less favoured group are likely to experience poorer life chances. Where there is poor or limited social mobility, a person's life chances are more likely to be affected by factors beyond their control because they are structurally disadvantaged.

Access to good quality education, early intervention to support and promote children's development, and ensuring that good quality health and care services are available to all are often proposed as the best ways of overcoming bad life chances.

See also – Agency; Causality; Demography; Epidemiology; Inequalities

Further reading

Marmot, M. (2016) *The Health Gap: the challenge of an unequal world*. London: Bloomsbury.
Wilkinson, R. and Pickett, K. (2010) *The Spirit Level: why equality is better for everyone*.
    New York: Bloomsbury.

Loss

The term 'loss' is frequently used in discussion, debates and conversations about experiences such as grief and bereavement. Grief is the emotional response to loss and can be experienced as a profound feeling of deprivation from losing someone or something. Bereavement is the state of loss.

A person may experience bereavement and a grief reaction when a relationship ends because a person dies or leaves the relationship. This may be a temporary loss or a permanent separation from someone to whom they have an emotional attachment. A sense of loss may be felt when a person is not, and can no longer be, physically present. It can also be felt when something less tangible and more abstract, such as romance or an employment status that is highly valued and perhaps a part of an individual's identity, is lost.

Losses can be multiple and related. For example, illness may lead to unemployment, which might lead to divorce and the loss of a person's home. The cumulative effect of losses such as these can trigger mental ill health. This is particularly the case where loss(es) impact on a person's identity and cause their status to change. In these cases a person may need to adapt to a new lifestyle or circumstances, and adjustment difficulties can follow.

Nurses and other health and social care workers often come into contact with individuals who have experienced loss. It is always important to identify the significance of any loss for the person experiencing it. There is a strong chance that the experience of loss can disrupt or unsettle a person's sense of self and security or 'world view', making them vulnerable to psychological and mental health difficulties. On the other hand, the experience of loss can also lead to positive change if an individual's adjustment and adaptive abilities allow or enable this. Viewing the world differently, taking new opportunities and constructing a new, fresh sense of identity can be liberating and empowering for some people, when the initial pain of their loss has subsided.

See also – Attribution theory; Empathy; Memory; Mental health; Resilience; Stress (and coping)

Further reading

Murray Parkes, C. and Prigerson, H.G. (2010) *Bereavement: studies of grief in adult life*, 4th edition. Harmondsworth: Penguin.

Market

The concept of a market is widely used in social science but has its origins in economics. It refers to a system or set of social relations that enables and facilitates the process of exchange. Essentially, a market is a place or means through which products and services can be bought and sold.

The concept of a market is usually associated with the forces of supply and demand. One party (the seller) offers their goods or services in exchange for money or something else of value to another (the buyer) who wishes to obtain them. Economists see the market as a device through which the price for goods or services is established. Markets also enable the allocation and distribution of goods and services within a society.

Supply and demand are the key factors that enable a market to operate. Demand for a product or service results from the extent to which consumers are willing to pay for it. Supply is the quantity of goods or services available from producers. Supply is affected by the cost of producing or providing goods and services. The lower the cost, the higher the supply and vice versa, generally.

The provision of services such as health and social care has been affected by 'marketisation' since the early 1990s, whereas the government or state provided most health and social care services before this point. This was a public sector monopoly where state organisations such as the NHS dominated healthcare provision. Critics argued that this led to a lack of choice in service provision, higher costs and poorer quality services because there was no competition between providers, as there would be in a market situation. Since the early 1990s governments have tried to introduce market mechanisms into both health and social care sectors by encouraging and supporting voluntary and private organisations to become providers of these services. Consequently, in some areas of care provision, such as nursing and residential home care for older people, the state has largely stopped being a direct provider of services. Private and voluntary sector organisations now dominate this part of the care market.

There are ongoing debates about the extent to which market ideas are appropriate or effective in the provision of health and social care services. For example, critics of private healthcare services argue that it is very difficult for potential consumers to assess the quality of care provided by different providers in their area. This undermines the notion of there being 'true competition' between providers. Similarly, high demand for health and social care services can't be managed by simply increasing the 'price' of the goods on offer to reduce demand. There is a moral and ethical requirement to provide health and social care services on the basis of need rather than the ability to pay. Despite this, marketisation of health and social care provision is likely to remain, in order to promote choice, maintain efficiency and raise quality through competitive pressures.

See also – Capitalism; Marxism

Further reading

Giddens, A. and Sutton, P.W. (2017) *Essential Concepts in Sociology*, 2nd edition. Cambridge: Polity Press.

Marxism

Marxism is a political and sociological perspective based on the work of Karl Marx (1818–1883).

Marx provided an account of the new class-based society that emerged after the Industrial Revolution. The Marxist perspective questions the functionalist idea that modern capitalist society is based on consensus (agreement) between the various social groups in society and harmony between social institutions. Instead, Marxists argue that society is really based on the unequal distribution of economic power and wealth.

Marxists believe that there are basically two social classes in capitalist societies, such as the UK. These consist of the bourgeoisie who own the 'means of production' (factories, land, etc.), and the proletariat who sell their labour to the owners of the means of production for wages. Marxists believe that the capitalist, bourgeois class exploit the proletariat and wield both economic and cultural power over them. This leads to a society that is characterised by antagonism and 'class conflict'.

Sociologists who use a Marxist perspective argue that the interests of the bourgeoisie are pursued at the expense of the proletariat, and vice versa. Marx himself argued that the bourgeoisie partly controlled society by developing and enforcing what he called a 'ruling ideology'. This is a 'package of ideas' that protects and approves the interests of the bourgeoisie. For example, the belief that everyone can achieve success by working hard, that wealth is the best measure of success and that business owners and 'bosses' are morally entitled to keep profits for themselves are part of the ruling ideology in capitalist societies.

Marxist sociologists argue that by accepting a 'ruling ideology' the proletariat doesn't act in its own interests and is oppressed by a 'false consciousness' – a failure by members of the proletariat to recognise their real interests. According to Marxism, revolution and a system of state controlled services would produce a better society that worked in the interests of everybody rather than just for the benefit of a privileged, powerful bourgeois minority. For Marxists, society functions to keep the bourgeoisie in power and the proletariat in a subservient position. From this conflict perspective, society is organised to ensure that this relationship continues and that class conflict is minimised.

Weaknesses of the Marxist perspective

Marxism offered a powerful, radical alternative to the functionalist perspective and was widely used in sociology in the 1960s and 1970s. However, contemporary sociologists are likely to criticise the Marxist perspective because it:
- puts too much emphasis on social class, and class conflict in particular
- doesn't recognise how employers and employees in modern societies do have shared interests in the success of a business or organisation and that both 'sides' are often happy to cooperate
- focuses on the economy as the driving force of social behaviour and ignores other important influences such as gender, ethnicity and religion, for example
- doesn't recognise that people are socially active with some power and the ability to make choices and influence the direction of their own lives.

See also – Capitalism; Functionalism; Sociological perspective

Further reading

Haralambos, M. and Holborn, M. (2013) *Sociology Themes and Perspectives*, 8th edition. London: Collins Education.

Maslow's hierarchy of needs

Maslow's hierarchy of needs is a model of human motivation based on the gradual satisfaction of different types of human need.

Abraham Maslow (1943) was interested in motivation and the way this affects human behaviour. He wanted to show that humans are not blindly reacting to situation or stimuli, as behaviourism implies. He believed that a person's behaviour and development are needs-driven.

Maslow's humanistic approach to development and behaviour is based on the belief that human beings have a number of different types of 'need' and that these needs must be met or satisfied in a particular sequence before the person can develop further. Specifically, a person's basic physiological needs must be met

first before they can satisfy their safety and security needs. Their behaviour will then be motivated by a desire to satisfy their love and emotional needs. When these are satisfied, the person will be motivated to meet their self-esteem needs. At this point, the individual is in a position to focus on achieving their full potential or need for self-actualisation.

Maslow's contribution to the humanistic perspective focuses on the way in which human behaviour and development are motivated by distinctly human qualities and needs.

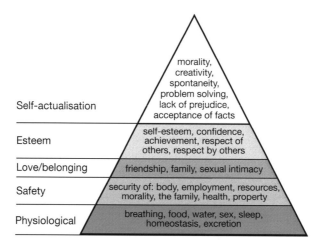

Figure 9 – Maslow's hierarchy of needs. Adapted and reproduced under a Creative Commons Attribution-Share Alike 4.0 International Licence. Author: Saul McLeod.

See also – Humanistic perspective; Self-actualisation

Reference

Maslow, A. (1943) *Motivation and Personality*. New York: Harper and Row.

Medicalisation

Medicalisation is a sociological term used to describe the process through which areas of social life have come under the medical gaze and have been 'colonised' by the medical profession.

Sociological critics of biomedicine use the concept of medicalisation to object to, and challenge, the expansion of medicine's social field of interest and power base. They argue that, throughout the twentieth and into the twenty-first century, the medical profession has sought to apply medical knowledge to a range of non-biological areas of social life and experience. Areas such as ageing, childbirth, children's behaviour and substance misuse have all become the focus of medical 'expertise' and have been redefined as medical 'problems'. The recent 'discovery' of attention deficit hyperactivity disorder (ADHD) as a medical disorder provides a good example of medicalisation. Some present-day medical practitioners believe that ADHD results from a biochemical disorder within the child, while others point to the way in which medical diagnosis judges a child's behaviour according to social criteria of what is acceptable and 'normal'.

White (2009) argues that through the medicalisation process, doctors use the power of biomedicine to construct new medical realities out of previously non-medical situations. For example, childbirth has largely become a clinical safety issue since being medicalised whereas it was, for much longer in human history, a natural process controlled by women. Feminist critics of the medicalisation of childbirth argue that the real purpose and effect of medical dominance in the area of childbirth is to define and control women's roles and social experiences (Oakley, 1979; Ehrenreich and English, 2005).

See also – Biomedical model; Feminism; Gender; Power; Social model of health

References and further reading

Coxon, K., Scamell, M. and Alaszewski, A. (2017) *Risk, Pregnancy and Childbirth*. Abingdon: Routledge.

Ehrenreich, B. and English, D. (2005) *For Her Own Good; two centuries of the experts' advice to women*. New York: Anchor Books.

Oakley, A. (1979) *Women Confined: towards a sociology of childbirth*. Oxford: Blackwell.

White, K. (2009) *An Introduction to the Sociology of Health and Illness*, 2nd edition. London: SAGE Publications.

Memory

Memory is a mental function that involves the encoding, storage and retrieval of information. It is an important concept in cognitive psychology and is widely understood in popular discourse as a key feature of human functioning.

Memory can be seen in terms of an information-processing system. Within this approach, the brain is the key memory processor that operates short-term (working) and long-term memory components. The information-processing approach to memory identifies three main stages of memory formation and retrieval:

1. Encoding – this involves the receiving, processing and combining of information received
2. Storage – this involves creating a record of encoded information in short- or long-term memory
3. Retrieval – this is the recall of stored information in response to a cue or stimulus.

The brain plays a key role in the information-processing approach to memory. By acting as a sense organ it acknowledges and responds to chemical and physical stimuli. Working memory makes sense of the stimuli and enables the person to respond. Long-term memory is the person's data store where they retain information and experiences and can draw on or recall them when necessary.

There is an extensive psychological research base and literature on the nature, functioning and use of human memory. In addition to studying normal memory, psychologists and other social scientists have studied the ways in which memory can be disrupted and damaged. Memory failure is often due to poor encoding, poor consolidation because memories 'merge' or become confused with other memories, or because retrieval cues are insufficient. Additionally, recall is disrupted, and memory formation can be prevented, by brain damage, disease, intoxication and drug use. Memory function can also be impaired by stress and anxiety and psychological traumas that cause memories to be repressed. Diseases such as stroke, Alzheimer's and other neurological conditions tend to lead to memory impairment too.

Effective memory is key to social functioning. The ability to make memories from experience and to recall them from short- and long-term memory enables a person to function socially. Everyday tasks in the home, basic travelling and work activity all rely on functioning memory. Nurses often have to support or find ways of helping people who experience memory problems with basic self-care and social functioning skills. The use of reminiscence therapy in residential settings for older people is an example of this. Similarly, when carrying out assessment of risk and mental capacity, memory function is always addressed and forms an important part of these assessments. Counselling and psychotherapy also focus on recall and revisiting of often painful memories. The aim is to reframe and restructure or contextualise memory to promote better mental health.

See also – Cognitive development; Cognitive perspective; Psychological perspective

Further reading

Baddeley, A., Eysenck, M.W. and Anderson, M.C. (2014) *Memory*, 2nd edition. Hove: Psychology Press.

Mental illness

Mental illness is a biomedical, psychiatric concept that is used to define, explain and understand experiences of mental morbidity and distress.

The concept of mental illness is controversial and disputed. Some health and social care practitioners do see mental health problems as a form of 'illness'. Others, using psychological and social perspectives, argue that an 'illness' approach is inaccurate and unhelpful in understanding the emotional and psychological difficulties or problems that people diagnosed with forms of mental illness experience.

Diagnosis of 'mental illness'

The psychiatric diagnosis of mental illness is similar to the diagnosis of physical health problems. Practitioners of both psychiatric and physical medicine tend to look for evidence of 'abnormality' within an individual. However, where practitioners of physical medicine carry out examinations, tests, X-rays and other scans to identify objective signs of physical 'abnormality' (high blood pressure, unusual pulse rates, 'abnormal' biochemistry results, tumours, fractures, bruising and bleeding, for example), psychiatrists can't directly see mental 'abnormality'. The 'mind', unlike the physical anatomy of the body, can't be

located or directly observed. As a result, psychiatric practitioners look for patterns of behaviour and subjective 'symptoms' (low mood, poor sleep, loss of appetite, lack of energy, unusual or distressing thoughts) to diagnose 'mental illness'.

Particular combinations of symptoms are believed to equate to different 'mental illnesses'. A number of mental illness classification systems exist. The International Classification of Diseases (ICD) system is probably the best known and is widely used by psychiatrists in the UK.

The power of the psychiatric perspective is such that its illness framework is often taken for granted as a valid and helpful way of understanding mental distress. It is widely used by general and mental health professionals as well as by members of the public as a language for thinking and talking about experiences of mental distress in contemporary society. As a result, the influence of general practitioners, psychiatrists and other care practitioners is powerful in determining what is and what is not considered to be a mental health problem. These people can define experiences and behaviour as evidence of

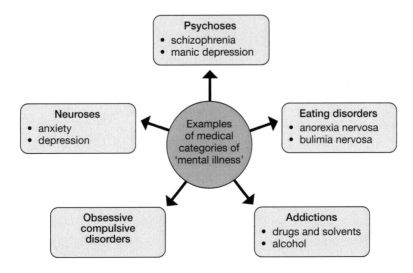

Figure 10 – Examples of medical categories of mental illness.

illness, and their expertise and authority are likely to be called on to confirm the opinion of lay people that their relative, friend or colleague has 'gone mad' (Rogers and Pilgrim, 2014).

Is 'mental illness' a myth?

Thomas Szasz (1961) first contested the claim that physical and mental illness are similar phenomena. Despite being a psychiatrist himself, Szasz argued that the term 'mental illness' is an inappropriate description of the mental distress that people experience. Instead, Szasz viewed 'mental illness' as a socially constructed myth maintained by the psychiatric profession. This is a controversial claim, given the widespread use and acceptance of psychiatric definitions of 'mental illness'. Szasz (1971) argued that mental distress is not the result of 'disease' or objective abnormality in the way that physical illness is. He argued that people who are diagnosed as suffering from 'mental illness' are really experiencing 'problems in living'. These are essentially social problems, not biomedical problems. Szasz saw 'mental illness' as a metaphor, not a 'fact'. He saw it as a way of dealing with people whose behaviour, beliefs and thoughts 'violate certain ethical, political and social norms' (Szasz, 1974, p. 23). As a result, Szasz (1974) saw the institutional, organised forms of psychiatric care as being repressive, coercive and performing a social control function in modern society. He argued that the role of the psychiatrist was to impose and police socially acceptable 'reality'. People who didn't accept, fit in with or exhibit conventional or acceptable forms of thinking, behaving and perceiving reality were, in Szasz's terms, deprived of their liberty and human right to self-determination by psychiatry.

It is important to note that Szasz (1974) and other critics of psychiatry are not denying the existence of mental distress or trying to say that psychological and emotional problems are not important features of human health and wellbeing. They are saying that these experiences aren't, from their perspective, 'illnesses' in the way medical practitioners claim they are.

See also – Anti-psychiatry; Biomedical model; Discourse; Psychiatry; Social model of health

References and further reading

Cromby, J., Harper, D. and Reavey, P. (2013) *Psychology, Mental Health and Distress*. Basingstoke: Palgrave Macmillan.

Rogers, A. and Pilgrim, D. (2014) *A Sociology of Mental Health and Illness*, 5th edition. Buckingham: Open University Press.

Szasz, T. (1961) *The Myth of Mental Illness*. New York: Hoeber-Harper.

Szasz, T. (1971) *The Manufacture of Madness*. London: Routledge & Kegan Paul.

Szasz, T. (1974) *Ideology and Insanity*. Harmondsworth: Penguin.

Migration

> Migration is the movement of people from one geographical location to another, usually across the borders of nation states and often between continents.

Migration has become a global social, political and economic issue in the early twenty-first century. However, the mass movement of people from Africa and the Middle East to Europe, as well as the movement of people from eastern to western Europe, is only one example of the large-scale migrations that have happened throughout history. Mass migration is, in fact, responsible for the spread of human beings across the world. Social scientists identify major social changes such as industrialisation, urbanisation and globalisation as drivers of migration. In addition to war and famine which tend to be 'push' factors, economic opportunities and political freedom are major 'pull' factors drawing migrants from one place and society to another.

Cultural and ethnic diversity are the main social consequences of mass migration. The increase in intensity of global migration since the Second World War has changed the ethnic composition of many European countries. Typically, this has involved the emergence of minority ethnic communities in larger cities in the countries of destination. Castles (2007) has identified four different models of post-1945 mass migration:

- The classic model – encouraging immigration to develop a country's economic capacity and offering eligible migrants citizenship (e.g. Australia, Canada)
- The colonial model – periodically encouraging and allowing immigrants from former colonies to migrate and settle on a permanent basis (e.g. UK and France)
- The guest worker model – allowing migrants entry for a specific purpose and a limited time to meet labour market needs (e.g. Germany, Switzerland)
- The illegal migrant model – this occurs through illegal evasion of border restrictions and national laws. Refugees and economic migrants may seek to enter a country and live as 'illegal aliens' with the assistance of people smugglers (e.g. North America, UK).

Critics of migration theories such as those above question whether it makes sense to focus on nations and national population movements as the key elements of mass migration any longer. Shared ethnic, religious and cultural identities are now also relevant to understanding both the factors underpinning migration and the impact of it on the countries and communities of destination. Migration as a concept and issue has become a major issue within the social sciences. It is now recognised that because of long-term and ongoing migration processes, many societies are constituted by, and can be understood in terms of, migration at a deep level.

See also – Citizenship; Demography; Globalisation; Industrialisation; Urbanisation

Reference

Castles, S. (2007) Twenty-first-century migration as a challenge to sociology. *Journal of Ethnic and Migration Studies*, **33(3):** 351–371.

Modernity

> Modernity is a historical period beginning in the mid-eighteenth century and lasting until the mid-1980s (or possibly later).

The beginnings of modernity coincided with the European Enlightenment of the eighteenth century. This describes a shift in thinking and social practices away from the received wisdoms of tradition, religious belief and the authority of the church towards scientific thinking and a drive for greater freedoms and equality in society. Sociology and other social sciences also developed during this period. They too challenged the traditions and historical restrictions of church and state and offered other ways of understanding and improving society during a period of huge social and political upheaval.

Modernity is the historical era in which sociologists identify capitalism, industrialisation, urbanisation, shifting class relations, the growth of democracy and the decline of religion as drivers and features of fundamental social change in society. A push for equality, and challenges to social inequality, came from a broad range of social groups (the working class, women, minority ethnic groups, etc.) during this period. Science became the key discourse in society, affecting production methods, education and the healthcare field, amongst others. Rational thinking and bureaucracy became the modus operandi of government, business and welfare organisations throughout society.

Modernisation affected many areas of social relations, social attitudes and aspects of society, from housing to politics, education and fashion, during the twentieth century. Many politicians, economists and sociologists saw modernity and modernisation processes as positive and progressive influences on western societies such as the UK, and believed this would spread to other non-western societies. The so-called 'modernisation thesis' maps out a process of economic, social and political development that moves a society from a traditional, agrarian stage to an advanced capitalist economy with progressive values and modern institutions. However, not all societies have followed this pattern. African and South American countries, as well as Japan and China, have modernised but not in a western way. This suggests there are multiple modernities rather than a single, linear route to modernisation.

Critics of the concept of modernity argue that it is too broad, vague and not very useful as an analytical tool. It describes rather than helps explain society and social change. Whilst describing a process of social development and economic growth, the concept of modernity also fails to account for the downside of modernisation. Arguably this includes socio-economic inequalities and financial instability in developed economies as well as the economic dependency of poorer nations on more developed nations. In these ways, modernisation is seen as a flawed concept. In response to these and other postmodern criticisms, sociologists such as Giddens (1990) argue that the negative consequences of modernisation are now recognised by social scientists and others as we progress through 'late modernity'. Facing up to social inequalities, environmental damage and the exploitation of economically poor but resource-rich countries by western nations and corporations is part of this. In addition, the continuing pursuit of gender and racial equality, the democratic redistribution of power and ensuring resources are shared more equitably remain important goals for those who see modernity as an unfinished project (Habermas, 1983).

See also – Postmodernism; Society

References

Giddens, A. (1990) *The Consequences of Modernity*. Cambridge: Polity Press.
Habermas, J. (1983) 'Modernity – an Incomplete Project', in H. Foster (ed.) *The Anti-Aesthetic*. Seattle: Bay Press.

Moral panic

A moral panic is an overreaction at a community or societal level towards a specific behaviour (e.g. glue-sniffing) or a group of people (e.g. gypsy travellers) that is seen as being symptomatic or representative of a wider social malaise or moral decline in society.

The concept of a moral panic emerged through the work of Stanley Cohen (1972). Cohen was interested in how deviant behaviour became amplified in society to the extent that it came to be viewed as a 'social problem'. Cohen's now famous study of youth cultures, *Folk Devils and Moral Panics* (1972), was based on his observations of minor altercations in Clacton between youths belonging to so-called rival Mods and Rockers subcultures. Cohen found it difficult to understand how what he had witnessed came to be reported and understood as a 'social problem'. He argued that 'youth' in general was scapegoated in exaggerated media reports about relatively minor incidents, to the extent that a 'labelling process' occurred and led to deviancy amplification. Cohen's concept of moral panic has been used to explore and explain how teenage pregnancy, community care of mentally ill people, dangerous dogs, 'legal highs' and ideas about immigrants and immigration have all been the focus of moral panic.

Cohen's (1972) study showed how the labelling of a group of people as outsiders ('folk devils') amplifies perceptions of deviance and stokes concern about what may be happening to society. A scapegoated group – 'youth' in this case – effectively takes the blame for social changes, subcultural behaviour or changing social practices that are experienced as unsettling, unwanted and a threat to 'moral values' or public safety. Media exaggeration of the apparent 'threat' occurs through sensationalised reporting. This draws public attention to the issue, amplifying the level of 'concern'. An increasingly alarmed public then demands 'action' from politicians, 'the authorities' and law enforcement agencies. Laws may be passed to ban the threat (raves, legal highs, a breed of 'dangerous dog'), initiatives introduced to 'tackle the problem' (better sex education for teenagers, better aftercare for people discharged from mental health units), or the attention of the media moves somewhere else.

The concept of moral panic is part of the interactionist approach within sociology. It focuses attention on the way interaction processes and 'meaning' can construct or make social realities. However, critics of this approach generally, and of the concept of moral panic in particular, argue that there are aspects of reality, such as terrorism, child abuse and climate change, that we should be worried about regardless of how much the media exaggerate their threat. As such, they suggest that the concept of 'moral panic' is too vague to help us distinguish between a real and an exaggerated threat to society. Despite this, the concept remains useful as a way of understanding how certain groups become stigmatised, marginalised and labelled as 'deviant' because they threaten the established sense of social order and provoke demands for social control to be imposed on them.

See also – Interactionism; Labelling theory; Stereotyping

Reference

Cohen, S. (1972) *Folk Devils and Moral Panics: the creation of the Mods and Rockers*. London: MacGibbon and Kee.

Mortality and Morbidity

Mortality

Mortality refers to death.

Social scientists study the rate of mortality, the social and economic determinants of mortality rates and how societies respond to death. There is a large, mainly statistically-based literature on the links between mortality and socio-economic factors within the social sciences. Social scientists have consistently argued that patterns of health and illness experience and death rates are not naturally occurring or the result of chance but are socially patterned. Large-scale and longitudinal data analyses have shown that the mortality rates are not evenly distributed across societies in the twenty-first century (Mackenbach, 2006).

Mortality statistics are compiled from information provided by doctors, who complete a death certificate when a person dies. Taken together, all of this information describes the social distribution of death in society. The statistics that are developed from analysing death certificates are sometimes referred to as 'death rates'. They indicate that there are social patterns to mortality.

In the early 1970s, the mortality rate among males of working age was twice as high for those in the lowest social class as for those in the highest. By the late 1990s, the figure was *three* times higher! This widening gap in mortality was caused by a faster decrease in mortality rates for more affluent groups in the population. In essence, a greater proportion of people in the higher social classes compared to those in lower social classes were living for longer. Mortality rates fell by 40% between 1970 and the late 1990s for social classes 1 and 2, by 30% for classes 3 and 4, but by only 10% for class 5 (the lowest social class; see *Table 10*). So, although death rates have fallen across all social groups and for both sexes in the late twentieth century, the difference in the expectation of life is widening between the more affluent and the poorer groups in society.

For men belonging to social classes 1 and 2, life expectancy at birth increased by two years during the 1980s; yet for classes 4 and 5, the increase was only 1.4 years. Men could expect to live to 75 in the higher social classes, but only to 70 in the lower classes. Women could expect to live to 80 in the higher social classes, but to 77 in the lower classes.

Table 10 – Registrar-General's social class scale

Social class number	Social class type	Types of occupation
Class 1	Professional occupations	Lawyers, doctors
Class 2	Intermediate occupations	Executives, shopkeepers
Class 3N	Skilled, non-manual occupations	Clerks, policemen
Class 3M	Skilled, manual occupations	Electricians, coal miners
Class 4	Partly skilled occupations	Farm workers, bus drivers
Class 5	Unskilled	Labourers, cleaners

Morbidity

Morbidity refers to levels of illness and disability in the population.

Morbidity data tends to be based on either the number or incidence of diseases, disabilities or injuries a person says they suffer or the amount of 'sickness' time they experience. Social scientists who investigate morbidity tend to be interested in quality of life and the impact that experiences of illness and disability have on individuals and society as a whole.

Unlike death rates, there does not appear to have been a decline in morbidity rates during the latter part of the twentieth and the early part of the twenty-first century. However, we should bear in mind the subjective nature of health and illness. Whereas mortality rates are based on the objective evidence of a certified death, morbidity data is often based on self-reported illness symptoms and claims of disability. This subjective data is less robust, as the criteria people use to define themselves as 'ill' or 'disabled' differ within

and across social groups. Bearing this in mind, the Acheson Report (1998) found that of those aged 45–64, 17% of professional men reported a 'limited long-standing illness' (sometimes referred to as 'chronic illness'), compared to 48% of unskilled males. For women of the same age, 25% of professional and 45% of unskilled women workers disclosed such a condition. This pattern of higher morbidity rates in the lower social classes affects not only experiences of physical health; it can also be seen that mental health problems are linked to social class (see *Figure 11*).

People with lower incomes, who are more likely to be in social classes 4 (semi-skilled manual) or 5 (unskilled manual) are significantly more likely to experience psychosis.

See also – Epidemiology; Life chances; Social class

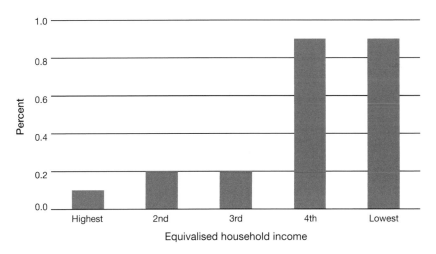

Figure 11 – Prevalence of psychotic disorder in adults in 2006 (age-standardised), by equivalised household income. Copyright © 2009, re-used with the permission of NHS Digital. All rights reserved.

References and further reading

Acheson, D. (1998) *Independent Inquiry into Inequalities in Health: report*. London: HMSO.
Mackenbach, J. (2006) *Health Inequalities: Europe in profile*. London: Department of Health.
Wilson, F. and Mabhala, M. (2009) *Key Concepts in Public Health*. London: SAGE Publications.

Motivation

Motivation is a psychological concept that refers to the energy or drive that sustains goal-directed human behaviour. The concept of motivation is also used to attribute reasons for behaviour or to explain the actions, desires and needs underpinning an individual's behaviour.

Motivation has a biological basis in terms of drives to meet basic needs (e.g. for food and shelter), to reproduce (sex drive) and seek pleasure. There are also social aspects of motivation, such as the drive or need to belong and to achieve.

Theories of motivation can be categorised as follows.

Instinct theories

These view motivation as having an innate, biological basis and argue that the instincts that drive human motivation are common to all people. But what are these instincts? It is not possible to produce a definitive list. Some people don't express these instincts (e.g. they are 'celibate') or can override them (e.g. anorexia). A person's instinctual motivations can also be disrupted by illness, disease and mental disorder.

Drive theories

This approach to explaining human motivation is based on the idea that humans are predisposed to seek a balance or status quo in terms of body and mind. From this perspective, primary drives relate to physical balance (e.g. shivering/sweating to maintain body temperature) and are automatic. Secondary drives refer to social and psychological motivations such as the drive to form friendships (i.e. to belong) or to achieve personal potential (self-actualise).

VIE/Expectancy Theory

Vroom (1964) developed the Valence, Instrumentality and Expectancy (VIE) approach to motivation to explain the complexities of human motivation. This approach, also known as Expectancy Theory, took understanding of motivation beyond the concepts of 'instincts' and 'drives'. Vroom argued that the strength of any motivation is defined by the way the following interact:

- Valence – how attractive is the action to a person? What reward will it bring?
- Instrumentality – the idea that performance of the action will lead to the reward
- Expectancy – the belief that exerting the effort needed will lead to a successful performance.

Vroom's (1964) VIE theory can be used to explain why we (and others) may choose to act in different ways in a given situation. We may choose to act (or not act) because of any of the VIE elements. We weigh up the likely outcome of our actions by how much we want it (at the time), how easy it is to act and how likely we are to achieve our goals.

Motivation is a significant issue for many people working in the health and social care sectors. For example, psychologists have focused on the way that motivational drives underpin, and can explain, the expression of some health-related (and unhealthy) behaviours and how psychological processes such as repression (a defence mechanism) affect the expression of motivated behaviour. Similarly, other psychologists and healthcare workers have found the concept of learned helplessness useful in understanding why some people appear to lack motivation of the desire and drive to change their behaviour. Nurses need to understand the origin of motivations affecting people's health-related behaviours, especially behaviours that have a detrimental effect on health and wellbeing. The use of motivational interviewing and strengths-based approaches to treatment and rehabilitation also draw on ideas about motivation, linking this to people's needs and capacities.

See also – Behaviour; Humanistic perspectives; Maslow's hierarchy of needs; Needs

Reference and further reading

Ryan, R.M. (2014) *The Oxford Handbook of Human Motivation*. Oxford: Oxford University Press.

Ryan, R.M. and Deci, E.L. (2017) *Self-Determination Theory: basic psychological needs in motivation, development and wellness*. New York: Guilford Press.

Vroom, V.H. (1964) *Work and Motivation*. New York: John Wiley & Sons.

Narrative(s)

> Narratives are stories or accounts that connect real or imagined events into a series of actions or experiences that have a collective and intentional coherence to them.

Understanding people's actions and experiences in narrative terms provides an explanatory framework for the social sciences. It is associated with qualitative and ethnographic research where lived experience, meaning and observation are seen as important in understanding the detailed, context-dependent and personal nature of social life.

Narratives tend to have 'themes' and may follow genre convention. People tell stories in various ways about themselves and others and the world(s) they occupy. Narratives both construct and communicate knowledge.

Narrative in social science is closely linked to psychology and human psychological functioning. People need, and are told or given, narratives to form their sense of personal and cultural identity. Memories are also constructed through the use of narrative. In this way we construct a sense of self through the stories we tell and that we are told about 'who' we are. These might include gender narratives (what it means to be a boy/girl, man/woman), narratives about 'race'/ethnicity and age, for example. Narratives help us to know who we are as well as providing a means of communicating this to others.

A person experiencing psychological distress/problems may be seen as experiencing a breakdown in their access to and use of a coherent, personal narrative. Repairing or reconstructing this narrative plays an important part in recovery.

Nurses should be aware of 'illness narratives' that people use and tell to make sense of their (ill) health experiences. Forms of illness narrative include:

- restitution – illness as a temporary disruption or detour from their story of normal life and health
- chaos – illness is seen as a permanent worsening state that damages and prevents a return to a preferred or normal life story
- quest – illness is an opportunity for transformational change, including psychological and spiritual renewal; the person's narrative recounts how they have, or will, overcome adversity.

Human beings create and tell stories to both communicate their experiences and understand or offer explanations of events. The narratives that people make and share provide an account of how and why events or experiences were or are generated. In this way narratives are central to cognitive or thinking processes and also provide a way in which the detail of human experience can be understood and communicated to others in society.

Narrative is linked to discourse, qualitative data, ethnographic approaches and a focus on lived experience in social science research. Narrative enquiry aims to uncover and analyse the detailed human stories and the way they are told and understood. Social scientists are often interested in exploring the links between institutional discourses (big stories) and the everyday, lived experiences of individuals and social groups (little stories) in order to analyse narrative production, practices and communication in society.

See also – Attribution theory; Discourse; Ideology; Memory

Further reading

Andrews, M., Squire, C. and Tamboukou, M. (eds) (2013) *Doing Narrative Research*, 2nd edition. London: SAGE Publications.

Riessman, C.K. (2008) *Narrative Methods for the Human Sciences*. Thousand Oaks, CA: SAGE Publications, Inc.

Need

A need is a necessity, something that a person requires to sustain or maintain an acceptable standard or quality of life. When a person's needs are not met, they will experience an adverse or negative outcome. This may involve ill health, disability or even death, if a person's basic nutritional or safety needs are not met.

Need is a fundamental concept in the thinking and practice of healthcare workers such as nurses. It may be used to identify and make sense of the basic, biological human requirements for life (e.g. food, water, air) or it can be used to help understand the social and psychological aspects of being human and the factors that motivate human behaviour.

Abraham Maslow's hierarchical model of human needs is widely known and used within health and social care practice, particularly in nursing. Maslow links human needs to motivation and behaviour, arguing that there is a hierarchy of human physical and psychological needs that drives behaviour. Maslow is typically viewed as a humanistic psychologist, although the approach that treats 'needs' as equivalent to drives is more often linked to behaviourism.

Conceptions and understanding of need can also vary between cultures and even between groups within a society. This leads social scientists to debate the extent to which human needs are universal or contingent on culture and other non-biological, socio-economic factors.

Doyal and Gough (1991) presented an approach to human need based on the argument that a person's needs represent 'the costs of being human within society'. A person whose needs are not met will function poorly with society. They argue that every person needs to possess physical health and personal autonomy to participate in the social setting in which they live. In addition to adequate physical health, it is argued that a person's capacity to make informed choices in life requires mental health, cognitive skills and social skills.

Doyal and Gough (1991) identify twelve categories of 'intermediate need' that define how needs for physical health and personal autonomy are fulfilled:
1. Adequate nutritious food and water
2. Adequate protective housing
3. Safe work environment
4. Supply of clothing
5. Safe physical environment
6. Security in childhood

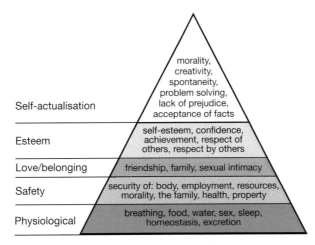

Figure 12 – Maslow's hierarchy of needs. Adapted and reproduced under a Creative Commons Attribution-Share Alike 4.0 International Licence. Author: Saul McLeod.

7. Appropriate healthcare
8. Meaningful primary relations with others
9. Physical security
10. Economic security
11. Safe birth control and child-bearing
12. Appropriate basic and cross-cultural education.

People use various ways of identifying and satisfying their own needs. However, those with more assets or capacities have more capabilities (choices, skills, freedoms) to achieve their needs and avoid poverty and ill health.

There is a great deal of ongoing debate about the nature, significance and role of 'needs' in human behaviour. Themes within these debates have focused on issues and questions such as:
• What should the standard of 'need' be and who should define it?
• How does the social and cultural consensus about what constitutes 'need' vary and change within and between societies and over time?

• How do individuals, activists and health and social care professionals define 'need' and to what extent do their definitions differ?

'Need' is a concept that is now deeply embedded in the organisation of health and social care services as well as in the thinking and practices of those who deliver care. The development of the welfare state in the mid-twentieth century led to a focus on meeting the 'needs' of those who most required healthcare and social protection services. Nurses and other health and social care workers now invariably assess and try to address people's unmet health and social support needs. As a consequence, 'need' is often a taken-for-granted concept used to explain what being human involves, as well as providing insight into the underlying motivation for human behaviour.

See also – Humanistic perspectives; Ideal type; Maslow's hierarchy of needs

Reference and further reading

Dean, H. (2010) *Understanding Human Need*. Bristol: Policy Press.
Doyal, L. and Gough, I. (1991) *A Theory of Human Need*. Basingstoke: Palgrave Macmillan.

Neuroscience

Neuroscience is the scientific study of the human nervous system, particularly the brain, and its impact on human life. It is an interdisciplinary area of study drawing on scientific disciplines including biology, physiology, physics, psychology, pharmacology and medicine.

Neuroscience was initially focused on understanding the brain as an anatomical structure and on tracing the impact that different aspects of brain structure have on human functioning and capabilities. It has become a much broader and more diverse discipline over the last 20 years, as it has been applied and extended to exploring molecular, cellular, developmental, evolutionary, computational and medical aspects of the nervous system. It is now an important approach to human psychology, exploring the way the brain and nervous system generally affect human behaviour(s). In particular, cognitive neuroscience has attempted to uncover and outline the ways in which psychological functions are rooted in and produced by neural (brain) circuitry. The development and use of powerful brain scanning and imaging techniques over the last 20 years has accelerated the development and work of neuroscience in many areas.

Critics of neuroscience argue that it has a reductionist approach, suggesting that complex social and psychological issues can be traced back (or reduced) to brain structure and activity. For critics, this negates the vital influence of culture, social structures and environment.

Neuroscience is increasingly used in mental health research and practice. It is sometimes presented with evangelical fervour as the way of truly understanding and locating the cause or source of mental health problems – in essence, they are rooted in or are traceable to 'broken brains'. The belief, or claim, of strong supporters of neuroscience is that eventually all mental illness will be identifiable in the biological substrate of the brain. Whilst many professionals working in mental health settings do see the brain as playing an important part in mental disorder and distress, the idea that 'broken brains' are responsible for mental illness is strongly disputed. Instead, the consensus view is based on the argument that interaction between the human brain and the environment, especially during an individual's developmental years during childhood and adolescence, is important. Consequently, it is important to avoid reducing the biological element of mental disorder to genetics as though mental illness is 'locked in' to a person's genome and is therefore unavoidable. Critics argue that neuroscientists, and their supporters, who do this are presenting a reductionist argument that seeks to explain away rather than account for the contribution that culture, environment and human conduct also make to human behaviour.

See also – Biomedical model; (The) Body; Cognitive perspective; Genetics; Science

Further reading

Barker, R.A., Cicchetti, F. and Robinson, E.S.J. (2018) *Neuroanatomy and Neuroscience at a Glance*, 5th edition. Chichester: John Wiley & Sons.

Bear, M.F., Connors, B.W. and Paradiso, M.A. (2015) *Neuroscience: exploring the brain*, 4th edition. Philadelphia, PA: Wolters Kluwer.

Obedience

Obedience is a concept explored by psychologists who are interested in social influences on human behaviour. It is linked to the study of authority and the role and impact of authority figures on people's behaviour. It is the link between authority figures and human behaviour that distinguishes obedience from:
- conformity, which is behaviour that aims to fit in with or match the majority
- compliance, which is behaviour that aims to fit in with peers or an 'in group'.

Stanley Milgram and Philip Zimbardo, both American psychologists, each carried out a now famous study into the way that authority can produce obedience.

Milgram's experiment suggests that obedience to authority is a normal human response and something that most people are unable to resist. His experiment deceived participants into thinking they were going to take part in a study about punishment and learning. It was, in fact, about obedience and how long they would accept and obey orders for. Participants were told they had to give an electric shock to a person in another room each time they got an answer wrong on a learning task, and that the shocks got more intense with each wrong answer. If the person resisted or was reluctant to administer the shock when it was due to be given, the authority figure/ researcher encouraged them further. The study found that people would obey orders even when the result of doing so seemed to pose a risk of severe harm occurring to others. The power of authority was such that it overrode moral ideas about not hurting others against their will.

Zimbardo's 'Stanford Prison experiment' was conducted in a mock prison environment. It found that people randomly assigned to 'guard' roles would obey orders to the point where their behaviour became aggressive.

The concept of obedience draws attention to the way that power and authority can impact behaviour, especially in situations where there is a power imbalance between those involved. This is particularly relevant to nurses who are often in situations where they have far more power than the vulnerable people who require their help. As such, it is important to be aware of the need to think critically about care practices and the regimes, processes and 'traditions' that can lead to the disempowerment and abuse of patients and colleagues because of the operation and impact of authority.

See also – Agency; Authority; Behaviour; Power

Further reading

Gross, R. (2014) *Themes, Issues and Debates in Psychology*, 4th edition. London: Hodder Education.

Operant conditioning

> Operant conditioning is a behavioural technique that is used to promote learning through the controlled use of consequences.

This aspect of behaviourism is associated with B. F. Skinner who used experiments with rats and pigeons to develop his instrumental learning theory. Skinner built a special box – now known as a 'Skinner box' – to facilitate the learning of new behaviours. The box contained a lever which, when pressed, released a food pellet or 'reward' to the rat in the box. After some trial and error, the rat learned that lever pressing had a consequence – it would be rewarded with food. Skinner believed that the reward reinforced the rat's lever-pressing behaviour and made it more likely that this behaviour would be repeated, or occur again, in the future. It is because the rat requires a 'reward' that reinforces its behaviour that this is also called instrumental learning.

Understanding operant conditioning

Skinner's theory of operant conditioning is based on the idea that learning takes place through reinforcement. Skinner identified two types of reinforcement:

- Positive reinforcement, where the consequences following a behaviour are experienced as desirable
- Negative reinforcement, where carrying out a behaviour removes something unpleasant.

It is important to know that negative reinforcement and punishment are not the same things. Punishment occurs when behaviour is followed by consequences that are unpleasant. For example, slapping a child who misbehaves is physical punishment for being 'naughty'. However, behaving well in order to avoid being sent to bed early is negative reinforcement. Negative reinforcement is used to make something happen, whereas punishment is used to stop something happening.

See also – Behaviour; Behaviourism; Classical conditioning; Reinforcement

Further reading

Gross, R. (2015) *Psychology: the science of mind and behaviour,* 7th edition. London: Hodder Education.

Paradigm

Social scientists use this term to refer to a pattern of thinking or a set of concepts, including theories, research methods, assumptions and claims, that are established and which represent the orthodox position and set standards for what is seen as legitimate in a particular field (e.g. medicine, nursing, etc.) of knowledge. In this sense, a paradigm is a set of ideas and ways of working that define a discipline at a particular period of time. Thomas Kuhn (1970), the leading historian of science, defined a scientific paradigm as 'universally recognised scientific achievements that, for a time, provide model problems and solutions for a community of practitioners'.

Since Kuhn, paradigms have been closely associated with scientific theory, practice and ways of knowing. He argued that scientific paradigms have been dominant in western societies since the Enlightenment and that science as a paradigm underpins much larger cultural frameworks for knowing and understanding social and cultural life. Kuhn argues that a dominant paradigm offers a common framework for knowing, investigating and explaining phenomena but can also limit our ability to 'think outside of the box' because it can exclude other ways of knowing and being. Critics of biomedicine, such as those who subscribe to homeopathic medicine, for example, argue that this disadvantages and excludes those with beliefs and values outside of the dominant framework.

Kuhn (1970) argued that sciences move through periods of normal science where an existing model of reality creates and sustains an orthodox, accepted approach to problem-solving and periods of revolution. During revolutionary periods the orthodox model is increasingly questioned and criticised to the point where there is a build-up of anomalies that can't be explained by the accepted, orthodox approach. A paradigm shift can then occur where alternative concepts, ways of thinking and ways of working provide more plausible, enlightening or effective ways of understanding an issue or area of science.

The dominant paradigms or ways of thinking in a society are often invisible to, or taken for granted by, those who live in that society. The dominant paradigm for understanding health issues in contemporary western societies is western scientific medicine, for example. Its theories, assumptions, claims and approaches are largely accepted *as reality* and are seen as providing standard, authoritative knowledge on health matters at present. However, orthodox biomedical approaches also have limitations and are strongly contested in areas such as mental health, where their weaknesses and limitations have led to the emergence of alternative, non-medical ways of understanding the experiences of mental health and ill health.

See also – Discourse; Ideology; Science

Reference

Kuhn, T. (1970) *The Structure of Scientific Revolutions*, 2nd edition. Chicago and London: University of Chicago Press, p. 44.

Patriarchy

Patriarchy is a system of male dominance over women in both specific areas of social life and society in general.

Patriarchy is a sociological concept introduced by Engels in his analysis of social relations under capitalism. Engels believed that capitalism led to inequalities in society generally, one aspect of which was the gendered distribution of power. In essence, a relatively small group of wealthy men used a variety of means (e.g. laws relating to the inheritance of male heirs only, male-only access to education and the professions) to favour men, particularly men like themselves, and keep women in a subservient, socially excluded position.

Patriarchy has become a core concept within feminism, particularly socialist and radical feminism, which sees power as a key element of gender relations. The feminist slogan 'the personal is political' captures the view that patriarchal influences and forces impact on women's lives at a deep level. Issues such as domestic violence, sexual harassment and the stereotypical treatment of women as sexual objects have been used to highlight how patriarchal attitudes and practices operate on and impact women's lives. Expectations about women's unpaid domestic and child-rearing roles in the family, the medicalisation of childbirth and popular notions of beauty and 'feminine behaviour' are seen as products of patriarchal discourse and oppression that contribute to gender inequality. Feminist groups holding these types of views argue that the solution to patriarchy is to challenge and dismantle the patriarchal order and social institutions, such as the family, that perpetuate it.

Critics of the concept of patriarchy argue that it exaggerates men's power over women in society, pointing to growing and improving gender equality and changing social attitudes towards women over the last century. Despite this, women do generally have less status and receive lower pay than men in the labour market. They are also less likely to be in positions of power over men at work and in other social and political situations. Social scientists have also raised doubts about whether patriarchy can actually *explain* women's oppression. There is no indication in the concept of the mechanism(s) at work in the patriarchal oppression of women. Sociologists have also wondered whether, and if so how, patriarchy works alongside other social differences and divisions – such as class, 'race'/ethnicity, sexuality and age – in oppressing women. This is important, as women's experiences of social opportunities and social disadvantage vary. Those sceptical of the power of patriarchy argue that it is important to consider the way inequalities intersect to advantage some women and disadvantage others.

See also – Feminism; Gender; Inequalities; Intersectionality; Power

Further reading

Haralambos, M. and Holborn, M. (2013) *Sociology Themes and Perspectives*, 8th edition. London: Collins Education.

Perception

This psychological concept refers to the way in which sensory information is identified, organised and interpreted as a way of constructing and understanding what is happening in a person's environment.

Perception is a function of the human nervous system. Signals in the nervous system are the result of physical or chemical stimulation in the sense organs of the human body. Perception is the process that makes sense of these signals. In effect, we receive vast amounts of information through our eyes, ears, nose, sense of taste and touch as well as our body position. We need to make sense of this to understand where we are in the world, what is happening and how this affects us. We do this very rapidly by processing the stimuli via our nervous systems. The end result is a mental representation of what we see, hear, smell, taste or touch in the world around us at that time, for example.

Whilst perception is a complex, high-level process it is one that generally occurs without deliberate, conscious effort on the part of the individual. However, there is an ongoing debate about whether perception is an active process of hypothesis testing, checking stimuli against available information sources in the memory, or whether it is much more passive, relying on the automatic processing of stimuli that we can make sense of due to prior experiences.

Perception tends to become an issue for nurses when a person presents with some form of perceptual disorder. This can occur as a result of:

- neurodegenerative disorders (e.g. dementia)
- acquired brain injury (including stroke)
- autism (i.e. sensory processing disorder)
- mental illness (e.g. hallucinations)
- substance misuse.

Dysfunction in one or more of a person's senses or in the ability of their brain to process sensory stimuli may cause a range of difficulties that affect their ability to function and can be very disabling.

See also – Biomedical model; Neuroscience; Psychiatry; Psychological perspective

Further reading

Gross, R. (2015) *Psychology: the science of mind and behaviour*, 7th edition. London: Hodder Education.

Rogers, B. (2017) *Perception: a very short introduction*. Oxford: Oxford University Press.

Personality

The concept of personality is widely used and understood in popular culture. It tends to be seen as the combination of characteristics and qualities that make up an individual's character. It is associated with other concepts such as identity, psyche and character.

Psychologists view personality as a set of individual differences that distinguish one person from another. An individual's personality is both characterised and influenced by their values, attitudes, memories, social relationships, upbringing and habits. There are a number of different theories of personality. Some of these focus on specific aspects of personality whereas others address the concept of personality and the process of personality development much more broadly. These include:

- biological theories
- behavioural theories
- psychodynamic theories
- humanistic theories
- trait theories.

Biological theories see personality as being rooted in a person's genetic inheritance. In essence, they argue that we inherit personality characteristics from our parents. Studies of twins have been widely used to test for similarities and differences in personality between twins brought up together and those who grow up apart. Those who grow up together should have very similar personalities because genetic or 'nature' and 'nurture' influences would be aligned. Those who grow up apart will only have similar personalities if genetics are a more powerful influence on personality development than nurture or environmental influences. Other psychologists, such as Hans Eysenck, have argued that biological processes such as cortical arousal can also affect personality. He claimed that high cortical arousal led to extrovert (outgoing) personalities whilst low cortical arousal led to introverted (quiet, shy) personalities because cortical arousal leads people to seek out stimulating experiences.

Behavioural theories focus on the way that personality is shaped through interactions between individuals and their environment. It says nothing about the origins or features of personality but does provide some ways of understanding why individuals' personalities develop in the way they do. In particular, they argue that our personalities are strongly influenced by the ways in which we learn and have our behaviours reinforced by others as we develop throughout the human lifespan.

Psychodynamic theories are based on the original work of Sigmund Freud (1856–1939). He developed the concept of the unconscious mind and argued that an individual's early experiences play a critical part in their psychological and emotional development. Freud described the human personality as a combination of the Id, Ego and Super-ego. He claimed that the Id controls and expresses an individual's needs and urges, whilst the Super-ego acts as the individual's conscience, imposing morals and ideals on the person. The Ego is the mediator between these other two aspects of personality, moderating the demands of the Id, the rules of the Super-ego and the realities of everyday life.

Humanistic theories focus on the concept of the self rather than on personality directly. Personality is seen as being an integral part of the self, which all people possess and seek to develop throughout their lifespan. Humanistic theorists argue that every individual has free will that allows them to make choices and decisions based on a personal assessment of their own best interests, wishes or preferences. Additionally, a person's experience of everyday life is individualised – no two people experience exactly the same things. As a result, our personalities are stimulated and developed through the ways we use our free will and respond to our particular experiences of everyday life. At the same time, it is argued that human beings have an innate, or inborn need to pursue self-actualisation. This means that people generally pursue opportunities for personal growth and development and that this need to achieve self-actualisation motivates a lot of our behaviour choices and the way we express ourselves. Carl Rogers and Abraham Maslow were prominent humanistic theorists who developed and applied many of these ideas.

Finally, trait theories argue that human personality consists of a number of broad 'traits'. A trait is a relatively stable personality characteristic that causes a person to behave in a particular way. Cattell (1957), one of the pioneers of this approach to personality, famously identified 16 human personality factors or 'traits' including: warm; abstract thinker; emotionally stable; dominant; enthusiastic; conscientious; bold; tender-minded; suspicious; imaginative; shrewd; apprehensive; experimenting; self-sufficient; controlled; tense.

He later narrowed this down to five big personality factors, summarised as OCEAN:

- Openness
- Conscientiousness
- Extroversion
- Agreeableness
- Neuroticism

Trait theories are used to explain how people relate to the world (including other people, e.g. as extroverts or introverts) and how they experience the world and themselves (e.g. neuroticism/stability). Trait theorists argue that an individual's unique personality results from the way in which these personality traits combine.

See also – Humanistic perspective; Identity; Psychodynamic perspective; Psychological perspective

Reference and further reading

Cattell, R.B. (1957) *Personality and Motivation Structure and Measurement*. New York: World Book Co.

Gross, R. (2015) *Psychology: the science of mind and behaviour*, 7th edition. London: Hodder Education.

Person-centred counselling

> Person-centred counselling is an approach to psychological intervention and support that puts into practice a range of concepts and techniques developed by humanistic psychologists and practitioners.

The goal of person-centred counselling is to support and enable the individual to develop a sense of self that gives them insight into how their attitudes, emotions and behaviours affect the way they relate to others and experience the world more generally. Carl Rogers' person-centred approach to counselling is now widely used and very influential in the health and social care sector. Rogers (1961) identified the three conditions of genuineness, empathy and unconditional positive regard as fundamental to effective therapeutic communication.

- Genuineness involves being yourself and contributing to interactions and relationships with honesty and integrity. Health and social care workers who are genuine in their interactions avoid being authoritarian, defensive or professionally detached.
- Empathy involves the ability to see and experience situations from another person's perspective.
- Unconditional positive regard involves accepting and validating an individual's experiences, feelings, beliefs and judgements unconditionally and in a non-judgemental way.

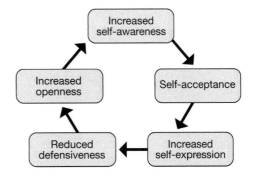

Figure 13 – The goals of person-centred counselling.

Non-judgemental acceptance of people enables health and social care workers to connect with the real, unique people they care for and support. Similarly, those who use a person-centred approach to counselling use genuineness, empathy and unconditional positive regard to help the person they are working with develop a positive self-image and greater self-acceptance.

See also – Empathy; Humanistic perspective; Rogers, Carl; Self-concept and Self-esteem

Reference and further reading

Mearns, D., Thorne, B. and McLeod, J. (2013) *Person-Centred Counselling in Action*, 4th edition. London: SAGE Publications.

Rogers, C. (1961) *On Becoming a Person: a therapist's view of psychotherapy*. Boston, MA: Houghton Mifflin.

Personalisation

Personalisation means that "every person who receives support, whether provided by statutory services or funded by themselves, will have choice and control over the shape of that support in all care settings" (Department of Health, 2007).

Personalisation has its origins in the independent living campaigns of the 1970s disability movement. Disability campaigners at the time advocated a social model of disability based on the values of empowerment and choice. The disability movement resisted institutional living and the controlling 'expertise' of professional practitioners such as doctors, nurses and social workers, for example. Disability movement critics felt that recipients of care were treated as passive and were made to fit in with existing services. Independent living required much more personalised provision, ideally chosen by the individual. As a result, disability services have gradually moved away from a care-based approach to a support-based style of provision in which the individual has much greater control and choice in relation to their support and the way(s) it is provided. As a fundamental principle underpinning this change in approach, personalisation guides health and social care practitioners to find ways of ensuring that the person with support needs has as much choice and control over their support as they want or are able to accept.

The Social Care Institute of Excellence (SCIE, 2010) captures much of the debate about, and goals of, personalisation when it suggests that in practice it means:

- tailoring support to individual needs
- ensuring people have access to information, advocacy and support to make informed decisions
- finding new ways of collaborative working so that people can be actively engaged in the design, delivery and evaluation of services
- having leadership and organisational systems that enable staff to work in person-centred ways
- embedding intervention, reablement and prevention
- ensuring a 'total system response' whereby all citizens have access to universal community services and resources.

In effect this means that personalisation has required health and social care service providers to shift the way they think about their role and the strategies they've previously used to provide services. In particular, they must now view individual needs and ways of meeting them from the perspective of the service user. In the past, services were created and made available and people were referred to them assuming that there would be a match between service provision and user need. If not, the individual's needs would remain unmet, or perhaps be only partially met. With the introduction of personalisation, health and social care providers now have a responsibility to find, or create/co-produce, services that work best for the person. Changes to the way in which services are funded have been used to facilitate this shift in focus and power away from service providers to service users. Funding strategies such as self-directed support, personal budgets and direct payments to service users are all designed to facilitate the personalisation agenda. Service users eligible for these forms of funding are now in a position to commission their own packages of care and support.

Personalisation is generally seen as a progressive development that, in moving power away from service providers to service users, provides people with a more appropriate, individualised and flexible way of obtaining the types of care and support they want. However, critics of personalisation argue that it:

- is overly individualistic and a threat to the collective provision of care and support services

- can lead to greater inequality in access to services as not everybody wants or is able to take responsibility for commissioning or managing their own care and support
- has been, or is being, used as a way of creating a privatised market in care services that undermines public sector (e.g. local authority and NHS) provision
- has not resulted in public sector services being redesigned to make them more flexible and personalised

- results in the costs of, and responsibility for, service provision being shifted to service users who find themselves with sources of funding (e.g. personal budgets) that are often insufficient to meet their particular care and support needs.

See also – Agency; Autonomy; Life chances; Power; Professionalism

References

Department of Health (2007) *Putting People First: a shared vision and commitment to the transformation of adult social care.* London: DH.

Social Care Institute of Excellence (2010) *Personalisation: a rough guide.* London: SCIE.

Phobias

A phobia is an intense, irrational, specific fear of an object, situation or event that, in reality, poses little or no danger.

The term phobia is sometimes used in everyday, popular language to convey a dislike of, or desire to avoid, a situation, object or person ('He's a bit computer-phobic') but this is an inaccurate and misleading use of it. A person may be diagnosed with a phobia by a medical or mental health practitioner or by a clinical psychologist if their irrational fear and avoidant behaviour is dysfunctional and disrupts their normal life. A diagnosis may then be given if the person's fear (of open spaces, confined spaces or social situations, for example) is unfounded, causes them severe and persistent distress and has a negative, detrimental effect on their everyday behaviour and functioning. Obtaining a diagnosis is necessary before a referral for treatment can be made to psychiatric or psychological services.

Phobias are anxiety-based disorders that can be effectively treated with cognitive behavioural therapy or behaviour modification techniques such as systematic desensitisation. This involves reducing and ultimately removing the power of a maladaptive association by gradually exposing the person to the thing they are frightened of. To do this the care practitioner and the phobic person first create a 'hierarchy of fear'. The treatment stage involves gradually exposing the person to varying degrees of fear whilst also helping them to relax and cope with each exposure. The goal is for the person to face the situation or object that they are fearful of or phobic about, without worrying. Systematic desensitisation has been used effectively to help people overcome all kinds of phobias, from agoraphobia (fear of open spaces) to arachnophobia (fear of spiders), that cause distress and disrupt people's lives.

See also – Anxiety; Behaviour modification; Cognitive behavioural therapy; Mental health; Post-traumatic stress disorder

Further reading

Cromby, J., Harper, D. and Reavey, P. (2013) *Psychology, Mental Health and Distress*. Basingstoke: Palgrave Macmillan.

Gross, R. (2015) *Psychology: the science of mind and behaviour*, 7th edition. London: Hodder Education.

Piaget, Jean

Jean Piaget (1896–1980) was a Swiss psychologist who pioneered the cognitive approach in his work on children's thinking and learning. Piaget believed that children's thinking and intelligence developed over time as a result of biological maturation. He developed a stage-based theory of cognitive development in which each stage of intellectual development built on a previous one.

Table 11 – Piaget's stages of cognitive development

Stage	Age (years)	Focus of development
Stage 1 Sensorimotor	0–2	The world is experienced via motor activity and the senses
Stage 2 Preoperational	2–7	Language develops with memory, the child is egocentric and unable to conserve (i.e. to think logically)
Stage 3 Concrete operational	7–11	The child can understand conservation (the ability to think logically) but can't solve problems mentally
Stage 4 Formal operational	11+	The child can use abstract thoughts and represent problems or 'see' them at a mental level in their thoughts

Piaget's theory claims that cognitive development occurs when the child's brain has matured so that it is 'ready' for development. He argued that new information and experiences are gradually assimilated into the child's existing thinking. When this happens, new experiences are accommodated by modifying existing thinking.

See also – Child development; Cognitive perspective; Psychological perspective

Further reading

Doherty, J. and Hughes, M. (2013) *Child Development: theory and practice 0–11*. Harlow: Pearson.

Gray, C. and MacBlain, S. (2015) *Learning Theories in Childhood*, 2nd edition. London: SAGE Publications.

Postmodernism

Postmodernism is a recent and quite controversial perspective in sociology. As its name suggests, this perspective is based on the idea that modern industrial society, in which social institutions, social roles and the beliefs people held were relatively clear and straightforward, is now in the past. Postmodern society is much less stable, more fragmented and fast-changing. It makes no sense to talk or think about 'the Family', for example, because family structure and people's roles and relationships within them are diverse. Similarly, in employment situations there is no longer a 'job for life' or a predictable career path available to most people. Working life – like social life in general – is seen as much less certain, more fragile and risky.

Postmodernists argue that society is not based on stable, relatively permanent social institutions that people can base their lives around. Instead, society is much more individualised and based on temporary associations between people and short-lived structures. People are no longer 'trapped' by their gender, ethnicity or social class – they are free to make their own decisions, to invent and reinvent a lifestyle that suits them. As a result they are less likely to see themselves as part of larger social groups with shared goals and interests, such as 'the working class' or 'liberal feminists', for example.

One of the key characteristics of postmodernism is its rejection of attempts to devise or present single, all-encompassing explanations of the social world. These all-encompassing theories are often referred to as 'grand narratives'. Examples include Marxist social theories, which claim that social class relations are the key factor that can lead us to the 'Truth' about the organisation and operation of society.

Postmodern social thinkers, on the other hand, tend to adopt a more relativist, subjective approach to the social world. As a result, postmodernism sees the role of sociological thinking as the recognition and acceptance of the rich diversity of beliefs, experiences and perspectives that exist in society. Postmodernists claim that the contemporary social world is characterised by disintegration, uncertainty, eclecticism, cultural democratisation and the questioning of 'expert' knowledge and authority. Postmodernist social thinkers argue that this shift away from accepting 'certainty' towards 'relativism' should be celebrated because it allows us to rethink outdated explanations and approaches to the social world and alerts us to new possibilities for social organisation and activity.

Traditionally, the sociological and other physical and social science theories employed by healthcare practitioners have tended to be based on a number of 'universalist' ideas. That is, there has been an acceptance that human beings have universal 'needs', that people have similar health experiences at particular life stages and that we share 'health' goals. Postmodernism is quite effective, however, in drawing attention to the possibility that these 'universal' assumptions are now inadequate. For example, postmodernist thinkers are likely to argue that traditional social and physical science disciplines overlook the specific dimensions of 'need' that are significant for particular individuals and cultural groups. Postmodernism is effective in pointing out that, as healthcare practitioners, we may be working with distorted or 'blunt' notions of social identity and human 'need'. In this way it has contributed to a concern with identity and the cultural aspects of health experience as well as raising the visibility and significance of marginalised social groups and their health concerns.

Despite the possibilities that post-modernism offers for the critique and rethinking of our 'traditional' sociological understanding of healthcare practice and experience, it has always aroused considerable controversy within the sociology and healthcare communities. One of the main criticisms of postmodernism as an approach to sociological thinking is that it lacks a political dimension. That is, it is useful as a way of critiquing or 'deconstructing' other ideas and theories – it is a good way of 'clearing the ground' – but it doesn't actually lead us towards any particular social goal. Postmodernism rejects the idea of social 'evolution' and 'progress' through increasing rational understanding of the social world. It seems to be apolitical in this sense and to ignore the need for social transformation. This can infuriate sociological thinkers who point to the existence of social inequalities and their impact on people's lives and believe that sociological data can inform social and healthcare policies that may make the social world a more equitable and equal place.

See also – Social action and social structure; Sociological perspective; Sociology

Further reading

Butler, C. (2002) *Postmodernism: a very short introduction.* Oxford: Oxford University Press.
McDonnell, O., Lohan, M., Hyde, A. and Porter, S. (2009) *Social Theory, Health and Healthcare.* Basingstoke: Palgrave Macmillan.

Positive psychology

Positive psychology is a relatively new branch of, or approach to, psychology that focuses on positive aspects of human life such as happiness, wellbeing and flourishing (personal growth). This is in sharp contrast to the way that orthodox psychology has historically focused on mental dysfunction, psychological pathology and the shortcomings or flaws of people rather than on their potential. Psychology has, as a result, historically operated within a disease model.

Positive psychologists have identified the importance of social relationships with a partner, family, friendship group and wider social networks as being important in improving and maintaining happiness. Physical exercise and sufficient income also play a part in promoting happiness and a positive sense of wellbeing.

Positive psychologists focus on researching the role and impact of 'flow' (states of pleasure), values, strengths, talents and the way these can be promoted by social systems and organisations within them.

One of the key insights of this approach within psychology is that people are more motivated by the future than they are driven by the past. Positive psychologists view mental health as a combination of high emotional, psychological and social wellbeing and low mental illness.

Positive psychology interventions aim to promote and sustain strategies for living well, achieving potential and enhancing wellbeing. It is constructive and proactive in its attempts to prevent problems developing and in seeking to solve problems in ways that make use of the person's strengths to achieve change and self-fulfilment. It plays a part in rehabilitation and recovery processes where healthcare workers seek to engage and build up a person's motivation to overcome difficulties or change problematic health behaviours (e.g. addictions). Positive psychology techniques and ideas also feature in the way healthcare workers are supervised and mentored to promote their personal and professional development.

See also – Mental illness; Psychoanalysis; Psychodynamic perspective; Psychological perspective

Further reading

Boniwell, I. (2012) *Positive Psychology in a Nutshell: the science of happiness*, 3rd edition. Maidenhead: Open University Press.

Post-traumatic stress disorder (PTSD)

Post-traumatic stress disorder (PTSD) is a mental health problem experienced by people who have been exposed to traumatic and frightening events. Typically, this includes soldiers, victims of crime and people who have suffered serious abuse.

An individual diagnosed with PTSD will become emotionally distressed and often very frightened when a stimulus that reminds them of the traumatic event (a car backfiring = gun fire, an unexplained noise downstairs = burglar, for example) causes them to re-experience it. As a result, people with PTSD are often very anxious, have poor sleep and poor concentration and may be hyper-vigilant (extremely watchful and alert to danger) because they believe the event could recur. This may lead to them using avoidance strategies, becoming withdrawn and estranged from others, and developing maladaptive feelings and behaviours, as ways of coping.

Mental health workers who support and treat people diagnosed with PTSD try to get them to make new associations (about the event and its consequences), reframing their thoughts in a way that leaves the traumatic event in the past. The goal is to ensure that the person doesn't feel the events are recurring. Classical and operant conditioning techniques are combined in this kind of behavioural treatment. They remove the association between fear-inducing stimuli and the past event whilst also minimising and controlling the physiological effects of fear, panic and anxiety through systematic desensitisation.

See also – Biomedical model; Mental illness; Psychiatry

Further reading

Regel, S. and Joseph, S. (2017) *Post-traumatic Stress: the facts.* Oxford: Oxford University Press.

Poverty

Poverty refers to the lack or scarcity of a needed resource. Social scientists have paid considerable attention to income poverty and the impact that a lack of money and material possessions can have on the health, wellbeing and life chances of individuals, families and social groups in society.

Social scientists make a distinction between absolute and relative poverty. Absolute poverty is defined as a point or standard of living beneath which a person experiences destitution. That is, they have insufficient resources (income, shelter, food) to meet their basic survival needs. Individuals and families living below the absolute standard of poverty face starvation and malnutrition. Relative poverty refers to having insufficient resources to achieve the minimum standards of living in a particular society. In essence, an individual has insufficient resources compared to others in society to the extent that they are excluded from social activity.

Social scientists (and government) may identify a numerical level or threshold to define both relative and absolute poverty. For example, a person who is living on an income of 60% or less of the median income in a given year is defined as being in relative poverty by the UK government.

In addition to having a low income and not being able to afford basic necessities, people are also sometimes asked by poverty surveys whether they subjectively consider themselves 'poor'. People who appear to have sufficient income can fall into this category when their debts, financial commitments and living costs are high and leave them without sufficient income to afford basic necessities.

The causes of poverty are widely debated and disputed. Some argue that the behaviour of individuals, families and social groups (including attitudes to work, values in relation to saving/spending and welfare benefit dependency) leads to poverty. On the other hand, the impact of the economy, social structures and restricted opportunities (including discrimination) are also used to argue that poverty can be produced by social factors that are beyond the control of the individual.

See also – Social class; Social policy; Underclass; Welfare

Further reading

Haralambos, M. and Holborn, M. (2013) *Sociology Themes and Perspectives*, 8th edition. London: Collins Education.

Lansley, S. and Mack, J. (2015) *Breadline Britain: the rise of mass poverty*. London: Oneworld Publications.

Power

Social scientists view power as a key resource in society. It is the ability to control, or at least influence, the behaviour of others. It can be used to control or enable the behaviour, activities and choices of individuals, social groups or the population as a whole. Power is seen as having both positive uses to enable social action and negative, constraining uses to coerce and control people.

Social scientists have a deep and long-standing interest in the nature of power (what is it?), how power is distributed (who has it?) and its impact in society (how is it used?). There are some circumstances where power that is seen as legitimate and given with consent (such as through elections) is used to create and impose collective rules, laws or other requirements on people or to make decisions on behalf of the population. These types of political authority and legal power do not necessarily involve the threat or use of force or violence but may do so where those in power feel it is necessary and justifiable to use the powers they have to protect the interests of the majority or their own interests.

These forms of so-called 'hard power' are rarely used in healthcare settings, though examples of coercion can be seen in mental healthcare when people are detained against their will, forcibly given medication or other treatments that they do not want or are physically restrained or secluded to prevent them behaving in ways that are seen as threatening or dangerous. 'Soft power', or the influence that comes from status and position and which is applied through relationships, is more widely used in healthcare settings. There are many unequal power relationships – such as those between practitioners and patients and between and within teams of healthcare workers, for example. This type of relational power – where one party has power over another – is often taken for granted in healthcare settings. The distribution of power within and between occupational hierarchies, such as when medical practitioners lead multidisciplinary teams, make final decisions to admit, treat or discharge patients and dictate the work and approach of other professionals, is an example of relational power that impacts the way nurses work in healthcare settings.

Power is no longer seen as a form of 'top-down' control by elites in society. Social scientists, influenced by the work of Michel Foucault (1980), now see power as a much broader, more ubiquitous feature of society. Foucault argues that "power is everywhere … because it comes from everywhere". Power is negotiated and used in every transaction and interaction in society. Some people might have legitimate authority, whilst others take and use power illegitimately. Those who have power and authority imposed on them also have the power of resistance available to them. People have found and use many ways of creating power and making power work for them – from using violence, coercion and manipulation to using guilt, shame and manipulation or even charisma and knowledge – to achieve their goals and get what they want.

See also – Authority; Discourse; Obedience

Reference and further reading

Foucault, M. (1980) *Power/Knowledge: selected interviews and other writings 1972–1977*. New York: Random House.

Foucault, M. and Faubion, J.D. (ed.) (2002) *Power: the essential works of Foucault 1954–1984 volume 3*. London: Penguin.

Lukes, S. (2004) *Power: a radical view*, 2nd edition. Basingstoke: Palgrave Macmillan.

Prejudice

Prejudice refers to negative, and often hostile and rejecting, thoughts and ideas about a person or group of people, based on insufficient knowledge and understanding. Prejudices often draw on and sustain stereotypes.

Prejudices are often learnt in childhood or are acquired through socialisation into a family, peer, work or subcultural group. They provide a way of marking out the boundaries of a group, enabling members to distinguish between people 'like us' and others who are outside of a group. Prejudices based on race, gender, social class, age, sexual orientation, religion and appearance are very common and underpin discriminatory behaviour. Unfair discrimination occurs when a person acts upon their prejudices. There are a wide variety of ways in which this can happen, including both overt and covert use of prejudice, that can result in behaviours that run from avoidance of certain others to genocide or the attempted wholesale destruction of a particular group of people.

Social scientists have generally focused on the way individuals develop and use prejudice in the way they relate to others. However, there is also some research into the way prejudices (e.g. about social class) relate to social structure and the life chances of larger groups within the population. Prejudice can underpin and justify exploitative social relations (e.g. in relation to gender equality) and can lead to discriminatory practices and policies (e.g. in the workplace or in pay). On closer analysis, prejudice is illogical, uninformed and counterproductive as it fails to assess individual capabilities, behaviour and needs. This is a key point or issue for all nurses as prejudice also denies people dignity as human beings and undermines equality and fairness.

See also – Attitudes; Discrimination; Stereotyping

Further reading

Dovidio, J., Hewstone, M., Glick, P. and Esses, V.M. (2010) *The SAGE Handbook of Prejudice, Stereotyping and Discrimination*. London: SAGE Publications.
Haralambos, M. and Holborn, M. (2013) *Sociology Themes and Perspectives*, 8th edition. London: Collins Education.

Profession

A profession is an occupational grouping that gives its members a status and reputation as having expertise based on training and the acquisition of a specialised knowledge base.

The concept of a profession is widely used but difficult to pin down. In current use, professions:

- are associated with giving public services in an impartial way that is beneficial to others and which is not motivated by self-interest
- tend to be autonomous and self-regulated rather than being directly governed or managed by employers; this is necessary for members of the profession to exercise their professional judgement independently
- generally have a licensing or registration system which members must be a part of in order to legitimately practise or claim membership of, as this regulates access to the profession
- set examinations of competence and enforce adherence to an ethical code
- are associated with occupations that give members special powers ('professional expertise') and prestige to the extent that they are seen as an elite group.

Doctors, lawyers, clergy, architects and the military are widely accepted as professions. Other groups, such as teachers, nurses and social workers, for example, have sought to achieve professional status but have not been entirely successful in doing so.

Critics of professions argue that:

- they have been seen by some as closed groups motivated by self-interest
- professional associations are seen as anti-competitive cartels that charge higher fees than necessary

- the status or prestige of professions has been undermined by celebrity culture and high salaries in the sport and entertainment industries
- professional status is no longer needed to achieve social and financial success in modern society.

There is some debate about the extent to which nursing has achieved, or can achieve, the status of a 'profession' such as medicine and the law. Most nurses are salaried, not self-employed, although they are governed and regulated by the Nursing and Midwifery Council and are required to work within a code of conduct that establishes and enforces professional ethics and standards. It is difficult to establish what professionally qualified nurses do that non-registered healthcare staff can't or don't do.

Social scientists generally view nursing (like social work and teaching) as a semi-profession on the basis that:

- training is shorter
- status and authority are lower than, say, medicine
- knowledge and expertise are less specialised
- individual practitioners have less autonomy – they are supervised and controlled by managers.

This does not mean that nurses do not show or use a professional level of dedication to patients, or that they do not strive for or achieve high standards of care or service for patients.

See also – Power; Role/role theory; Role models; Socialisation

Further reading

Dingwall, R. and Lewis P. (eds) (2014) *The Sociology of the Professions: lawyers, doctors and others*. New Orleans, LA: Quid Pro Books.

Susskind, R. and Susskind, D. (2017) *The Future of the Professions: how technology will transform the work of human experts*. Oxford: Oxford University Press.

Psychiatry

Psychiatry is a branch of medicine dealing with disorders in which mental or behavioural features are most prominent. Psychiatry provides a set of beliefs and concepts about emotional and psychological difficulties based on medical ideas of 'illness' and 'disorder'. These ideas, and the mental healthcare practices that result from them, are dominant within the statutory and private sector mental health systems in the UK and in developed, westernised countries generally.

Medically qualified psychiatrists tend to believe that mental illnesses originate from biological dysfunction. These include dysfunction of the brain, malfunctioning biochemical processes and the inheritance of 'faulty' genes that predispose people to mental illnesses. Psychiatrists who base their healthcare practice on biological psychiatry identify mental illness as being located within the individual who experiences mental 'distress' and exhibits symptoms of behavioural and/or emotional 'disorder'. Consequently, biologically orientated forms of psychiatry tend to underplay, and in more extreme cases ignore, the possible contribution and impact of other non-biological factors (cultural, social, psychological and spiritual, for example) in the causation of mental health problems.

Criticism of psychiatry

Critics of psychiatry challenge the medical claim that people experiencing mental distress have a mental 'illness' and that this is likely to be caused by factors within the individual (such as a 'broken brain'). There are many different critics of psychiatry who dispute the 'illness' approach to mental distress. These include the service user movement, mental health practitioners who use non-medical ways of understanding and explaining mental distress and academics who question the validity of 'mental illness' as a concept and claim it is a 'myth'.

See also – Anti-psychiatry; Mental illness; Social model of health

Further reading

Burns, T. (2006) *Psychiatry; a very short introduction.* Oxford: Oxford University Press.

Katona, C., Cooper, C. and Robertson, M. (2016) *Psychiatry at a Glance*, 6th edition. Chichester: John Wiley & Sons.

Szasz, T. (1961) *The Myth of Mental Illness: foundations of a theory of personal conduct.* New York: Hoeber-Harper.

Psychoanalysis

Psychoanalysis is mostly closely associated with Sigmund Freud (1856–1939), although it has been developed and practised since the late nineteenth century by a number of other theorists and practitioners (Jung, Adler, etc.). Psychoanalysis is both a set of theories about the structure and functioning of the human mind and an approach to psychological therapy. Psychoanalytical psychologists focus on the emotional and personality aspects of human development rather than on the learning or intellectual areas that cognitive theorists explore.

Psychoanalysis and personality

The word 'personality' comes from the Latin word 'persona'. This describes the mask worn during theatrical dramas. It refers to the relatively stable and enduring aspects of the individual that distinguish him or her from other people. Effectively, every human being develops a unique personality and identity. The development of personality is a dynamic and evolving process. Things are always changing and developing even though the qualities of an individual's personality remain relatively consistent over time.

Freud was interested in, and proposed a theory to explain, how human personality is structured and how it develops. Freud believed that the mind consisted of three 'territories'. These are the conscious; the pre-conscious; and the unconscious parts of the mind. The conscious mind is aware of the here and now, functioning when the individual is awake to behave in a rational, thoughtful way. The pre-conscious mind contains partially forgotten ideas and feelings. It also prevents unacceptable, disturbing unconscious memories from surfacing. The unconscious mind is the biggest part and acts as a store of all the memories, feelings and ideas that the individual experiences throughout their life. The things that lurk deep in the unconscious are seen to play a powerful, ongoing role in influencing the individual's emotions, behaviour and personality.

Freud also believed that the development and expression of an individual's emotions and behaviour are driven by the operation of what he called the Id, Ego and Super-ego. The Id is a raw mass of powerful, unruly energies that are pleasure-seeking and demand 'satisfaction'. The operation of the Id is unconscious but is continually seeking outlets. The Id is most powerful and is least checked when we are in our infancy. Newborn babies are completely dependent on others to satisfy their needs. The powerful, demanding Id causes the baby to kick and scream and react angrily when its needs aren't met immediately. The simple pleasure-seeking of the Id has to be controlled if the individual is to adjust to a society in which they are not the 'centre of the universe' and will have to compromise, share and accept that they can't always have what they want, when they want it.

The development of the individual's Ego begins when the child becomes aware that they will have to adjust their demands to fit in with the world around them. The Super-ego develops later when the child incorporates the standards of behaviour of people whose approval they value. The Super-ego is like the child's conscience, as it acts like an internal control on impulsive behaviour.

Psychoanalysis and psychosexual development

Freud's theories suggest that human development evolves as individuals progress through stages in which the basic instinctual sexual energy (called the libido) seeks expression in ways that are progressively more sophisticated. When Freud used the term 'sexual energy' he meant it in the broad sense of any pleasurable bodily sensation. This obviously includes the current, everyday use of the phrase but also refers to acts such as eating.

According to Freud, the greatest source of pleasure for a young infant is being fed. During feeding, particularly breast-feeding, the child's attention becomes focused on the person providing the nourishment. In most cases, this is the mother. Freud referred to early infancy (from birth to age one) as the oral stage of a child's development. This is when the baby's oral organs – lips, mouth and tongue – are its main means for obtaining the sensory (and 'sexual') pleasure of feeding. Freudian theory claims that a happy, balanced oral stage can tilt a child towards a happy adulthood. On the other hand, insufficient or excessive gratification during the oral stage can lead to psychological problems in later life. For example, over-indulgence can 'spoil' a child, resulting in an over-dependent adult.

During the second year of life, the anus and defecation become important sources of sensory (and 'sexual') pleasure for the child. Interactions between child and parents concerning toilet training take on special significance. It's at this time, from the age of one to three – the anal stage – that other adult predispositions are formed. For example, refusal to defecate when it's appropriate to do so can lead to obsessive cleanliness in adulthood. Toilet training routines cause the child to experience restrictions of the Id impulses but they also learn that they can challenge parental authority by rebelling against the training routine.

At around the age of three, the child enters the phallic stage, which lasts until age five. In this period, the child's genital organs provide the main source of sensory pleasure. During the phallic stage, children also develop a sexual desire towards the opposite-sex parent, and hostility towards the same-sex parent, who is seen as a sexual rival. Boys fall in love with their mother and resent their father, and girls long for their father and are jealous of their mother. This sexual attachment to opposite-sex parents and hostility towards same-sex parents is known, in the case of the boy, as the Oedipus complex, and, in the case of the girl, as the Electra complex. Faced with these powerful sexual urges, the child's mind does battle with its body's instincts. During the struggle, the Id (the impulsive instinct-driven part of the mind), is refereed by the Ego (the growing self-awareness of the mind). Out of the tug-of-war, the child, fearful yet loving of the opposite-sex parent, develops a Super-ego (the conscience of the mind).

The phallic stage is followed by the latency stage, lasting from around age six to puberty. During this time, child sexuality seems to lie dormant, and children concentrate on same-sex friendships. The genital stage comes next, beginning at puberty and lasting, more or less, for the rest of a person's life. Sexual interest is reawakened, and, for most people, the pursuit of opposite-sex partners is the norm. Freud viewed adolescence as the final stage of personality development that lasts for the rest of our lives but he also believed that 'the child within' never completely dies, as some of the drives from our oral, anal and phallic stages remain repressed in the unconscious, occasionally being expressed.

Freud believed that individuals who had difficulty in passing through any particular stage of psychosexual development will find this reflected in their adult behaviour and personality. Unresolved Oedipal conflicts may produce a person who has difficulty with authority figures and a poor sense of sexual identity. Anal personality types may show stubbornness, independence and possessiveness.

See also – Freud; Psychodynamic perspective; Unconscious mind

Further reading

Gross, R. (2015) *Psychology: the science of mind and behaviour*, 7th edition. London: Hodder Education.

Milton, J., Polmear, C. and Fabricius, J. (2011) *A Short Introduction to Psychoanalysis*, 2nd edition. London: SAGE Publications.

Psychodynamic perspective

The psychodynamic perspective focuses on the deep, inner psychological aspects of human development and relationships. It is strongly associated with the work of Sigmund Freud (1856–1939) and the treatment of 'abnormal' behaviour.

This psychological perspective was originally developed by Freud (1920) as psychoanalysis. Freud used his experiences as a therapist with mentally disordered people to develop key psychoanalytic ideas. He was particularly interested in the connections between abnormal behaviour and unconscious, underlying psychological processes. The psychodynamic perspective in psychology now covers more than Freud's original psychoanalytic ideas. Other theorists and practitioners developed and extended Freud's work throughout the twentieth century; Erik Erikson (1902–1994) was one of these people. Inspired by Freud's work, Erikson produced a theory of psychosocial development that has influenced the work of many psychologists, educators and health and social care practitioners.

The psychodynamic perspective suggests that unconscious forces and conflicts cause psychological disturbance. They are driven by memories, feelings and past experiences that are locked away in the unconscious but 'leak out' in dreams, slips of the tongue ('Freudian slips') and displacement behaviour. Early childhood experiences are seen as particularly important in creating unresolved psychological conflicts that become locked into the unconscious.

Table 12 – Evaluating the psychodynamic approach to health and social care provision

What does it offer?	What are its limitations?
Psychodynamic therapies are effective with certain types of people (articulate, introspective) and certain types of disorders (anxiety-based, linked to attachments and early experiences)	Psychodynamic therapies tend to focus on past experiences rather than the current difficulties a person faces
Psychodynamic therapies seek out the root causes of people's problems and try to resolve them	Digging deeply into a person's problems and past experiences can produce more distress (making the person feel worse) before a solution is found and symptoms are relieved
The psychodynamic approach can be used with individuals or groups	Psychodynamic treatment is costly and time-consuming and requires a specially trained therapist

See also – Defence mechanisms; Freud; Unconscious mind

Reference

Freud, S. (1920) *A General Introduction to Psychoanalysis*. London: Constable.

Psychological interventions

A psychological intervention is an action or strategy that is used to support or bring about change in a person's psychological functioning, behaviour or mental state.

Psychological interventions are most closely associated with mental health practice but may also be a part of the work and activities of other health, social care and education practitioners. Psychological interventions generally have the aim of relieving a person's psychological or emotional symptoms, changing their behaviour or uncovering and treating the cause of their distress or problems. However, psychological interventions that promote positive wellbeing, self-esteem, emotional development and happiness can also be developed and implemented by psychologists and other care, welfare and education practitioners.

The specific nature or form that a psychological intervention takes will depend on the psychological perspective that informs it. For example, a nurse trained in the use of cognitive behavioural therapy who is working with a depressed teenager will use different psychological interventions to a social worker supporting the parents of a child excluded from school because of behavioural problems. Psychological interventions need to be tailored to the specific needs of the individual and are most effective when there is clear consent from and collaboration with the person who experiences them.

See also – Behaviour modification; Cognitive behavioural therapy; Person-centred counselling; Psychoanalysis

Further reading

Gross, R. (2015) *Psychology: the science of mind and behaviour*, 7th edition. London: Hodder Education.

Psychological perspective

A psychological perspective is a distinct approach or school of thought within the broader academic discipline of psychology. Each perspective offers a particular way of looking at psychological issues or experiences based on the concepts, theories and research evidence they generate.

The main psychological perspectives within contemporary psychology are the:
- behavioural perspective
- social learning perspective
- psychodynamic perspective
- cognitive perspective
- humanistic perspective
- biological perspective.

Each of the main psychological perspectives has played an important role in the development of academic and applied psychology. They can be thought of as 'tools' in a toolbox that can be used to tackle different psychological challenges, although none of the perspectives is always best for every situation. Each approach has strengths and weaknesses and tends to be used to understand particular issues in human psychology.

See also – Behaviourism; Biological perspective; Cognitive perspective; Humanistic perspective; Psychodynamic approach; Social learning theory

Further reading

Glassman, W.E. and Hadad, M. (2013) *Approaches to Psychology*, 6th edition. Maidenhead: McGraw-Hill Education.

Gross, R. (2015) *Psychology: the science of mind and behaviour*, 7th edition. London: Hodder Education.

Public sphere

The metaphorical public space(s) where debate and discussion occur in contemporary society.

Social scientists contrast the public sphere with the private sphere. In communication terms, the public sphere includes newspapers, magazines, television programmes and the internet/social media sites that provide a democratic environment in which people can discuss, debate and share ideas and information. An active, accessible and unrestricted public sphere is seen as vital to democracy. Controlling, restricting and/or closing down the public sphere limits freedom and imposes authoritarian controls in a society.

Jürgen Habermas, a German sociologist, is most closely associated with social scientific work on the public sphere. He traces the origins of the public sphere to the eighteenth-century coffee houses and salons of European cities (London, Paris, Berlin, Vienna, etc.). Their development as a public sphere for debate paralleled the rise of mass media. This is now more closely associated with the concept of a public sphere, although Habermas argues that mass media and mass entertainment have stifled the public sphere and have resulted in stage-managed politics and narrower, more limited forms of democracy that are manipulated and controlled by a variety of commercial and other political and financial interests.

Critics of Habermas' claims about the decline of the public sphere as a democratic space argue that his notion of 'salon culture' was, in fact, socially selective and elitist. In particular, Habermas' public sphere seems to exclude the working class, suggesting that it was neither democratic nor accessible to all. This criticism can also be applied to women and minority ethnic groups. In fact, feminist critics of Habermas argue that the so-called 'public sphere' that he describes is, in fact, an example of how society is organised in a patriarchal way. The 'public sphere' is associated with and organised around the activities of men, whilst the 'private sphere' of the family and domestic home is associated with women. In this way, critics argue, the public sphere is an ideological device that legitimises social inequalities.

See also – Families; Feminism

Further reading

Calhoun, C. (ed.) (1993) *Habermas and the Public Sphere*. Cambridge, MA: MIT Press.
Haralambos, M. and Holborn, M. (2013) *Sociology Themes and Perspectives*, 8th edition. London: Collins Education.

Realism

> Realism is a philosophical approach or position used in social science research. The key claim of realism is that social reality is an objective phenomenon that exists 'out there' and can be accessed using scientific research methods.

Social scientists who take a realist position within their research investigations believe that knowledge exists in the 'real world' and can be discovered through observation and experience. As such, scientific research investigations enable us to get closer to the truth about social life. This contrasts with an idealist approach that argues knowledge is created in the human mind, through the way people think and attribute meaning to their experiences. Consequently, there is no pre-existing 'real world' to be discovered. It is made and remade through the ways people relate and interact and in the ways we negotiate and attribute meaning to our observations and experiences. This social constructionist approach has gained a great deal of support within the social sciences but has been countered by what is known as critical realism.

Critical realism is used within sociology to obtain objective knowledge of specific phenomena using scientific methods, whilst acknowledging that the knowledge obtained is contingent. This might include, for example, using data and knowledge from natural sciences and then assessing its validity and usefulness in the context of the social and historical situation or circumstances within which it is found. This challenges the social constructionist claims that there is no 'real world' and that all knowledge is produced or constructed through the actions and in the minds of social actors.

See also – Reflexivity; Social constructionism; Sociological perspective

Further reading

Burr, V. (2015) *Social Constructionism*, 3rd edition. Hove: Routledge.

McDonnell, O., Lohan, M., Hyde, A. and Porter, S. (2009) *Social Theory, Health and Healthcare*. Basingstoke: Palgrave Macmillan.

Reflexivity

Reflexivity describes both a thinking practice (a way of understanding) and a relationship between knowledge/knowing and the society or situation the person is in.

A person who uses reflexivity is reflective. As a social actor, they focus on how they are connected to, are impacting on and are affected by their social context. At the root of this concept is the claim that the self is constructed through social interaction. It is not innate but is an active, relational process. It is this process of 'self' construction that makes humans reflexive – we are engaged in social life whilst also being able to reflect on it.

Beck and Giddens both argue that in late modernity people are forced to reflect on their own lives and identities due to the collapse of 'tradition'. Beck refers to this stage in societal development as reflexive modernisation or the risk society.

Reflexivity is now central to social theorising and social research because the gap between the researcher and research subject is eroded. A social researcher can never be 'outside' of the social phenomenon they are investigating. There is no objective external world 'out there'.

Criticism

- Structural factors (e.g. class) still have a profound impact in shaping life chances/experiences. Individualisation thesis is exaggerated.
- Reflexivity in research can lead to self-indulgent reflections on the researcher's own thoughts about how they may be affecting the research process. As a result, the researcher can end up focusing more on their role in the investigation than on the aspect of social life they're studying.
- Reflexivity doesn't allow/validate large-scale social/attitude surveys (e.g. macro work) so we ignore/under-estimate patterns/irregularities that define 'society'.

Being reflexive involves considering your own place in the social world, not as an isolated and asocial individual but as someone who both contributes to, and is affected by, the 'greater-than-the-sum-of-the-parts' aspects of the human world. You contribute to the human-made aspects of world via your membership of different social groups and through participating in collective activities. However, your particular experiences of, and responses to, the social world also play a part in constructing and maintaining it. So, your experience of being a nurse is partly determined by the social role, status and expectations we presently apply to nurses. But it will also vary according to what age, gender, ethnicity, sexual orientation, nationality and social class background you happen to be. As a reflexive practitioner, you should be able to look 'outwards' as well as 'inwards' to understand how your own experiences, and those of your colleagues and service users, are historically located and socially situated. In doing so you will be 'thinking sociologically' and will be able to generate your own sociological understandings of nursing, or the healthcare field more broadly.

See also – Identity; Society; Sociology

Further reading

Beck, U., Giddens, A. and Lash, S. (1994) *Reflexive Modernization: politics, tradition and aesthetics in the modern social order.* Cambridge: Polity.

May, T. and Perry, B. (2017) *Reflexivity: the essential guide.* London: SAGE Publications.

Reinforcement

Reinforcement is a behavioural psychology concept that refers to any consequence that makes it more likely a person (or other non-human organism) will respond to a specific stimulus in a particular way.

For example, if a rat is given food for pressing a lever, it is more likely to press the lever again. In this case, food is used to positively reinforce the desired lever-pressing behaviour. Similarly, if a child is praised for desired behaviour, they are more likely to repeat that behaviour in future in order to receive praise again. In both of these examples, behaviour is being positively reinforced through rewards.

By contrast, negative reinforcement works in a slightly different way. Desired behaviour is more likely to occur because it ensures an aversive or negative consequence is prevented or postponed. For example, if a teenager really disliked being nagged by a very persistent parent to tidy their bedroom or turn their music down at home, they are more likely to do these things in order to avoid being nagged. The parent's nagging behaviour is the negative reinforcement in this situation.

See also – Behaviourism; Classical conditioning; Operant conditioning

Further reading

Gross, R. (2015) *Psychology: the science of mind and behaviour*, 7th edition. London: Hodder Education.

Research methods

Research methods are knowledge-production strategies that play a central part in social scientific exploration and understanding. Social scientists use research methods in order to:
- carry out exploratory research that helps to identify and define basic questions or research problems
- construct knowledge through testing theories and potential solutions to problems or questions that have been raised
- empirically test or validate the evidence for a claim, possible outcome or solution that has been proposed to a problem.

Social scientists tend to distinguish between qualitative and quantitative research methods. Some social science-based research studies employ both of these approaches in what is known as mixed methods research, although empirical research designs tend to have a leaning towards either qualitative or quantitative research methods. A social scientist will tend to select either a quantitative or qualitative research method in response to the nature of their research topic and the research question that they have produced.

Qualitative research methods tend to be used in exploratory, investigative studies that ask quite broad questions about human behaviour, meaning and experiences. Qualitative methods are also characterised by the use of non-numerical data such as word-based documents and texts, images and audiovisual materials. Typically, these studies are not seeking to measure variables or generate any quantifiable data or to establish the relationship between variables. Instead, they are more interested in 'rich', deep data and direct observation or participation in a setting that gives insight into how an aspect of the social world is experienced.

Quantitative research methods, in contrast to qualitative methods, do focus on producing and collecting numerical data in order to analyse and explain relationships between variables. As such, this type of research method tends to make use of a hypothesis that is then tested. Quantitative research methods require random samples of participants and use structured data collection instruments (such as questionnaires) that create a 'closed system' of predetermined response categories. This enables the research to summarise, compare and generalise from the data findings more easily.

Social scientists who use either quantitative or qualitative research methods to investigate areas that interest them, make use of primary and secondary data. Primary data is data that the researcher generates themselves as part of their research study. They may do this using questionnaires, individual or group interviews or through observation, for example. Secondary data, by contrast, is data that has already been generated by somebody else and which the researcher then makes secondary use of. This may be existing statistics, such as census or epidemiological data, case studies or audio/video recordings made by others that can be reanalysed from a new perspective or for a new purpose.

See also – Data; Hypothesis; Realism; Reflexivity; Sociology

Further reading

Ellis, P. (2016) *Understanding Research for Nursing Students*, 3rd edition. London: Learning Matters.

Lindsay, B. (2007) *Understanding Research and Evidence-Based Practice*. Exeter: Reflect Press.

Resilience

Resilience is a psychological concept associated with positive psychology. It refers to an individual's ability to draw on and apply the skills, abilities and knowledge they have acquired through education and experience to cope with and tackle the problems they face. In popular terms, it refers to the ability to 'bounce back'.

Definitions of resilience are wide and varied. Masten (2001, p. 228) argues that "resilience refers to a class of phenomenon characterised by good outcomes in spite of serious threats to adaptation or development". Carr (2004, p. 300) says something similar in suggesting that resilience is "the capacity to withstand exceptional stresses and demands without developing stress-related problems".

Resilience is often seen as the other side of the coin to vulnerability. However, it isn't just a static quality that a person has or hasn't got. Beardslee (1989, p. 267) acknowledges the way behaviours and thinking patters interact to produce resilience when defining it as "unusually good adaptation in the face of severe stress". Resilience is now most closely associated with the strengths-based approach to health and social care practice.

The concept of resilience has become more important in health and social care as practitioners have moved away from a 'needs-led' and problem-focused approach to care and support. Recovery-based approaches that focus on an individual's strengths and abilities rather than on their perceived deficits and problems focus attention on the positive qualities and capacities a person has for dealing with health, psychological and social issues that are affecting their quality of life and ability to cope. This is where resilience comes in!

Health and social care workers who adopt a resilience perspective encourage/motivate and support the people they work with to draw on the range of personal resources available to them in order to address their problems. These include the person's skills, abilities and knowledge as well as their social network (family, friendships and wider relationships). Realising that they have personal resources that can be used to improve their situation and that there are other sources of support (family, friends, neighbours) is a first step in using resilience. Developing new skills and trying out new experiences can also help people to strengthen and develop themselves in a positive, problem-solving way. This is more active and empowering than waiting for health and social care 'experts' to come up with a 'silver bullet' solution or treatment that will solve a person's difficulties. However, a resilience approach doesn't mean that an individual must take on sole responsibility for resolving their difficulties. It is better practice for health and social care workers to promote resilience through a partnership approach that:

- focuses on wellness, quality of life and recovery rather than illness
- recognises each person's individuality
- acknowledges the reality and impact of an individual's health problems or social care needs but doesn't see this as a reason to stop the person getting on with their life
- promotes and maintains a sense of hope and the expectation that the person can continue to enjoy, or regain, a good quality of life.

The resilience approach is now quite widely accepted and used in health and social care settings – especially where trauma, rehabilitation and recovery are important issues. However, the resilience approach is not above criticism. Those who do have reservations about it argue that the resilience approach, and the idea that everyone can develop resilience, doesn't always acknowledge the extent to which a person's illness or life trauma really can undermine an individual's capacity to cope and be independent. They also contend that it can be 'victim-blaming'. For example, are people who have little resilience not taking responsibility to get better or improve their circumstances? Should they just 'try harder'? Saying that a person 'lacks resilience' can sometimes involve blaming them when, in fact, the person lacks support – which is not their fault!

See also – Attachment; Empathy; Ethics; Personality

References

Beardslee, W.R. (1989) The role of self-understanding in resilient individuals: the development of a perspective. *American Journal of Orthopsychiatry*, **59**: 266–278.

Carr, A. (2004) *Positive Psychology: the science of happiness and human strengths*. Hove: Brunner-Routledge.

Masten, A.S. (2001) Ordinary magic. Resilience processes in development. *American Psychologist*, **56**: 227–238.

Risk assessment

Risk assessment is the process of identifying hazards and then evaluating the likelihood of a hazard actually causing harm. It is now a key feature of care practice for all health and social care workers. In practice, health and social care workers focus on assessing two types of risk:
- The risks a person poses to others (dangerousness)
- The risks a person is subject to (vulnerability).

In the majority of cases, health and social care workers are more likely to find themselves focusing on safeguarding and health and safety issues rather than the risks a person may pose to others. This is more a feature of mental health and some learning disabilities settings but does need to be taken seriously where it is an issue.

Hazards in care settings

Hazards in the physical environment of care settings include the following.
- *Faulty electrical appliances*, switches, overloaded sockets, frayed flexes and power surges can all lead to fires, burns and electrical shocks, for example.
- *Faulty gas appliances and gas leaks* can lead to fires, explosions, breathing difficulties, unconsciousness and asphyxiation.
- *Water leaks* result in wet floors, walls and carpets as well as rotten floorboards. All of these things cause accidents and injuries if people slip or trip. If there is contact between water and electricity there is also a danger of electrocution.
- *Kitchen hazards* include sharp knives, cooking appliances, pot handles hanging over edge of cooker, slippery floors, contaminated food.
- *Living room and bedroom hazards* include worn or badly fitted carpets, loose rugs, poorly placed furniture, floor-length curtains, clothes or bed linen left on the floor, trailing flexes, poor lighting, electrical appliances, fires without guards.
- *Bathroom hazards* include hot water, wet slippery surfaces and floors, electrical items near water.

- *Stairs* are hazardous if they lack hand rails, are steep or have poorly fitted, loose carpets.

Examples of care equipment hazards include:
- mobility aids that are the wrong size or which do not work properly
- faulty or damaged lifting equipment
- brakes and hydraulics on beds that do not work properly
- computer display screens and keyboards that are badly located, poorly serviced or over-used
- blades and syringe needles that are stored or disposed of incorrectly
- unlabelled, incorrectly labelled or leaking bottles and containers
- old and faulty electrical and gas-fuelled appliances
- excessively full or faulty waste disposal equipment.

Care practitioners should always check the equipment that they intend to use, to ensure it is safe and free of hazards. They should not use equipment that is faulty or which they have not been trained to use. Faulty, unsafe equipment should be reported and removed from the care setting.

The aim of risk assessment is to provide information that can be used to develop risk management strategies. These are ways of practising that reduce or minimise the likelihood of a potential hazard affecting the individual. The Health and Safety Executive has identified five stages of risk assessment (see *Table 13*).

Table 13 – The stages of risk assessment

Stage	Key questions	Purpose
Look for hazards	What are the hazards?	To identify all hazards
Assess who may be harmed	Who is at risk?	To evaluate the risk of hazards causing harm
Consider the risk – whether existing precautions are adequate	What needs to be done? Who needs to do what?	To consider risk control measures To identify risk control responsibilities
Document the findings	Can you give a summary of the hazards and risks?	To record all findings in the risk control plan
Review the assessment and revise if necessary	Is the risk controlled? Are further controls needed?	To monitor and maintain an accurate and up-to-date risk control system

The Management of Health and Safety at Work Regulations (1999) place a legal duty on employers to carry out risk assessments in order to ensure a safe and healthy workplace. The risk assessments that are produced should clearly identify:

- the potential hazards and risks to the health, safety and security of employees and others in the workplace
- any preventive and protective measures that are needed to minimise risk and improve health and safety.

Care practitioners can also carry out their own ongoing risk assessments in their everyday work. Basically this involves:

- being alert to possible hazards
- understanding the risks associated with each hazard
- reporting any health, safety or security concerns that are identified.

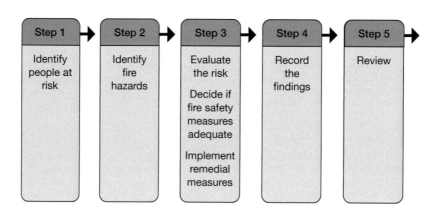

Figure 14 – The steps to take in carrying out a risk assessment related to fire hazards in a care home.

See also – Ethical issues; Self-harm; Violence

Further reading

Hart, C. (2014) *A Pocket Guide to Risk Assessment and Management in Mental Health.* Abingdon: Routledge.

Scott, M. and Fisher, M. (2013) *Patient Safety and Managing Risk in Nursing.* London: Learning Matters.

Rogers, Carl

Carl Rogers (1902–1987) was an American psychologist who is known as one of the pioneers of humanistic psychology. This focuses on the whole person and views each person as unique, rational and self-determining.

Rogers was very interested in the development of the self and made a considerable contribution to psychological understanding of human potential, the drive to grow and develop and the importance of enabling people to 'be themselves'.

Rogers (1963) was distinctive in the way he encouraged psychologists, educators and care practitioners to focus on and facilitate the capacity that people have for self-direction and for understanding their own development needs. Rogers noted that an individual's self-concept is strongly influenced by the judgements they make about themselves and by what they believe others think about them. For example,

a negative self-concept can develop if a person internalises critical comments that others make about them ('you're hopeless') and then thinks and acts as if this is true. Rogers was also concerned with the importance of self-esteem and the role of the 'ideal self' in the way that we make judgements about ourselves. Humanistic psychologists such as Rogers (1963) claim that a mismatch between the ideal self and actual self can lead to psychological and emotional problems.

See also – Humanistic perspective; Person-centred counselling; Self; Self-concept and Self-esteem

Reference and further reading

Gross, R. (2015) *Psychology: the science of mind and behaviour*, 7th edition. London: Hodder Education.

Rogers, C. (1963) *On Becoming a Person: a therapist's view of psychotherapy*, 2nd edition. London: Constable.

Role/role theory

The concept of role originated in sociology and is often referred to as a 'social role'. It refers to a set of behaviours, rights, obligations, expectations and beliefs that are associated with a particular social status and position (e.g. parent, policeman, teacher).

People perform multiple roles in their everyday life, depending on their relationship to others (as mother, father, brother, sister, grandchild, etc.) and their social situation (as employer or employee, student or professor, for example). Roles are therefore relational and also functional. Social learning theorists argue that social roles enable us to interact and behave in particular ways because we learn and 'perform' the behaviour and 'script' expected of that role (e.g. as student in relation to teacher). Roles also enable a division of labour to occur in society so that some people perform the role of doctor whilst others perform social work roles or nursing roles.

See also – Role models; Social learning theory

Further reading

Gross, R. (2015) *Psychology: the science of mind and behaviour*, 7th edition. London: Hodder Education.

Role models

Role models are people who inspire others to imitate or be like them because of their desirable characteristics. Bandura and Walters (1963) argued that we learn and develop through a process of imitating role models but that we also only imitate those behaviours we see as being in our interests.

The idea of modelling and learning through imitation has been used to promote anti-discriminatory behaviour and to persuade people to improve their health-related behaviours. Being anti-discriminatory and promoting health and wellbeing are key features of the care practitioner's role for many people working in the health and social care sectors.

Promoting anti-discriminatory behaviour and practices

A role model is somebody who is admired and whose behaviour and values are seen as desirable. Care practitioners tend to be committed to promoting equality and challenging discrimination in their everyday work. Expressing anti-discrimination values in the way that they relate to and interact with people and modelling behaviours that promote equality and fairness may encourage others (colleagues and people who use services) to imitate this kind of behaviour. In this way, the social learning perspective informs the approach care practitioners take in their care relationships.

Using positive role models in health education

Role models can use the influence they have over people who aspire to be like them to shape the health behaviours of the wider public. The concepts of role modelling, vicarious reinforcement and imitation have been widely used by health education campaigners to raise awareness of a range of health issues, including diet, exercise and breast cancer, for example, in ways that encourage people to change their behaviours. Diet, weight loss and healthy eating issues have been promoted by a range of celebrity chefs such as Jamie Oliver, Hugh Fearnley-Whittingstall and Gordon Ramsay over the past ten years. Similarly, television and radio chat shows and events such as the London Marathon frequently feature celebrities who are promoting health-related causes as a way of gaining wider publicity for them whilst also encouraging fans to change their health behaviour. The use of role models such as celebrities and sports performers in health education programmes is a deliberate attempt to draw on social learning principles.

See also – Humanistic perspective; Social learning theory

Reference

Bandura, A. and Walters, R.H. (1963), *Social learning and personality development.* New York: Holt, Rinehart and Winston.

Science

> Science is a method of knowledge production that tests hypotheses and theories against objective forms of evidence.

During the 'scientific revolution' that occurred in Europe in the seventeenth century, the term 'science' was used to describe a method of enquiry. In particular, it is associated with a systematic way of gathering data through observation and experimentation and the formulation and testing of hypotheses. By the nineteenth century it was used to describe disciplines that studied only the physical or material world, including physics, chemistry and astronomy. By the beginning of the twentieth century, the meaning of science had shifted to the methods that could produce valid and reliable knowledge of the physical, and increasingly the social and psychological, world.

The scientific method, and resulting knowledge, is often viewed as more rigorous and dependable than alternative forms of gathering knowledge, such as reflection. Nursing as an academic subject and area of healthcare practice draws on and applies a variety of science-based disciplines, including biology, chemistry and physics, to understand and respond to human health, illness and disease issues. The shift within nursing to evidence-based practice and the use of research data to inform and justify clinical interventions and nursing practice also illustrate the strong connection between science and contemporary nursing. However, there is also a tension within nursing between the use of objective, science-based theory and evidence and the importance of more intuitive, compassionate and experience-based responses to the human needs and essential humanity of each individual a nurse engages with.

See also – Biomedical model; Discourse; Ideology; Paradigm

Further reading

Holborn, M. (2015) *Contemporary Sociology*. Cambridge: Polity.
Smith, M.J. (1998) *Social Science in Question*. London: SAGE Publications.

Self

The self is an important concept used widely in the social sciences. It refers to an individual's awareness of having a distinct social identity.

The development of our sense of self is an ongoing, lifelong process. A newborn baby has no sense of self. An adult is far more aware of 'who' they are in a social and psychological sense because they have developed a deep understanding of how they feel and how they relate to and are perceived by others in the world. A person's internal or psychological sense of self connects them to their feelings and is the key source of self-knowledge or understanding. It is how we understand who we are as a person and both accounts for and explains what triggers much of our behaviour and the way we experience and respond to the situations and people we encounter. Social scientists also recognise that people also have an outer, social self that is presented to the external world. This is not a fixed sense of who we are but is flexible and adapted to respond appropriately to who we are interacting with at the time.

The ways in which people construct, experience and negotiate a sense of self in their efforts to understand and find a place in the social world is a major area of research and debate within the social sciences. Sociologists, psychologists and philosophers are all very engaged with issues of 'who am I?', what it means to be human and how the 'human condition' is experienced. However, Cromby et al. (2013) point out that the idea that each individual has, or is seeking, a 'unified self' is an assumption that is particular to western cultures and is central to the idea that people have (or should normally have) stable and coherent personalities. This assumption is incorporated into the way nurses and other healthcare workers focus on 'the individual' and seek to provide 'personalised' or 'individualised' care, for example. By contrast, people living in, or who have spent their formative years in non-western collectivist societies tend to have a sense of self that is more invested in community and family activities that are group- rather than individual-focused.

See also – Humanistic perspective; Identity; Psychological perspective; Rogers, Carl

Reference and further reading

Cromby, J., Harper, D. and Reavey, P. (2013) *Psychology, Mental Health and Distress*. Basingstoke: Palgrave Macmillan.
Elliott, A. (2013) *Concepts of the Self*, 3rd edition. Cambridge: Polity Press.

Self-actualisation

The concept of self-actualisation is commonly associated with Abraham Maslow's (1943) hierarchy of needs theory. It is the final stage, or ultimate level, of human psychological development – the actualisation of personal potential – that can only be reached when all of the individual's other basic and psychological needs have been met. Maslow's theory suggests that people have a psychological drive to achieve self-fulfilment and that a person must be making full use of their potential before they achieve this.

Carl Rogers (1902–1987), another humanistic psychologist, also argued that each person is born with a 'self-actualising tendency' – that is, a need to grow and develop to their full potential. However, people may develop a self-concept or have expectations and demands imposed on them that do not fit with their self-actualising tendency. Because they spend time and energy trying to conform to these expectations and demands, Rogers suggests that people in this situation will remain unfulfilled and unable to achieve their true potential.

The idea that human beings are predisposed to seek self-actualisation is not accepted by all social scientists. It is argued, for example, that some people make the mistake of seeking to actualise or perfect a self-image or ideal sense of self that they desire and wish to present to others.

This is not the same as achieving their potential. Similarly, critics of Maslow have argued that his claim that self-actualisation can only be achieved once other needs are met is mistaken. This kind of linear process may not apply, for example, when a person is unwell or disabled in some way and requires assistance to meet their needs whilst remaining capable of achieving other aspects of their intellectual or artistic potential. In addition, critics of Maslow and Rogers have pointed out that they do not consider the influence that a person's material circumstances and the opportunities available to them can have in either advantaging or disadvantaging them in their pursuit of self-actualisation.

See also – Humanistic perspective; Maslow's hierarchy of needs; Rogers, Carl

Reference

Maslow, A. (1943) *Motivation and Personality*. New York: Harper and Row.

Self-concept and Self-esteem

Self-concept

> Self-concept is an idea developed by those using a humanistic psychological perspective. A person's self-image combines with their self-esteem to make up their self-concept. An individual's self-concept is a central part of their identity. Having a clear, positive picture of who you are (self-image) and how you feel about yourself (self-esteem) helps to give you a sense of psychological security and affects the way that you relate to other people.

The self-concept becomes more sophisticated as we progress through childhood. Children move from being able to give surface, external descriptions of themselves to being able to describe their own internal qualities, beliefs and personality traits. They also become capable of making global judgements about their self-worth and self-esteem. Self-concept does affect a person's emotional and social development throughout the lifespan. For example, it can motivate us to do or try things (at school, at work or in our personal life) or stop us from seeking or taking opportunities.

Self-esteem

> Self-esteem refers to a person's sense of their self-worth. A person's self-esteem consists of beliefs ('I am kind', 'I am useless', 'I am unlovable', 'I am beautiful') about themselves, as well as emotions (pride, shame, sadness, happiness) that the person feels about themselves. In essence, self-esteem is a judgement that expresses what we think and feel about our 'self'.

Psychologists generally see self-esteem as a core, enduring feature of an individual's personality and a factor that influences motivation and attainment in a person's education, work and personal life. An individual with positive or high self-esteem is, for example, thought to be more likely to be happy, achieve well and feel fulfilled in their personal life and relationships. By contrast, a person with low self-esteem is thought to be more likely to be self-critical, pessimistic and envious of others. Self-esteem plays an important part in humanistic psychology.

See also – Humanistic perspective; Maslow's hierarchy of needs; Self

Further reading

Gross, R. (2015) *Psychology: the science of mind and behaviour*, 7th edition. London: Hodder Education.

Self-harm

The concept of self-harm refers to any form of deliberate self-injury that is intentional but not suicidal. Skin-cutting and self-poisoning are the most common forms of self-harm. Other less common forms include hair-pulling (trichotillomania), opening up cuts and wounds to prevent healing (dermatillomania), burning, scratching or hitting body parts and swallowing objects or toxic substances. There is usually a deliberate attempt to cause tissue damage in any form of self-harm. Adolescents and young adults are most likely to self-harm but self-harm does occur in all age groups.

Self-harming behaviour can be life-threatening and may have unintentionally fatal consequences. Some people do self-harm without having a diagnosed mental health problem. However, self-harm may also be a symptom of other conditions such as depression, eating disorder, post-traumatic stress disorder, anxiety disorder or borderline personality disorder.

People give a variety of reasons for self-harming. For example, some people use self-harm as a way of coping with extreme stress, intense anxiety, depression, feelings of failure or a deep sense of self-loathing and low self-esteem. A person's self-harming behaviour may be linked to traumatic events that have happened to them – such as child abuse, sexual assault or traumatic loss – or may be linked to ongoing patterns of dysfunctional or destructive behaviour such as perfectionism, addiction or self-image problems. People who present with self-harm injuries at Accident and Emergency departments have often consumed excessive amounts of alcohol prior to self-harming.

There are a number of different forms of treatment and support for self-harm, including:

- drug treatments, especially if self-harm is linked to anxiety or depression
- teaching avoidance techniques that aim to occupy the person with other activities when they are stressed and likely to self-harm
- harm-minimisation approaches, such as needle exchanges for heroin addicts, that aim to reduce the risk involved in some self-harming behaviours
- cognitive behavioural therapy that challenges dysfunctional thinking and destructive patterns of behaviour and equips the person with alternative ways of thinking and behaving
- relaxation/mindfulness techniques that aim to reduce underlying tensions and help the person to avoid stress and situations that may trigger their self-harming behaviour.

See also – (The) Body; Loss; Mental illness

Further reading

Chaney, S. (2017) *Psyche on the Skin: a history of self-harm*. London: Reaktion.

Separation (and loss)

Separation anxiety refers to the distress shown by an infant or young child when separated from his or her mother and the degree of comfort and happiness when reunited.

John Bowlby (1907–1990), a British psychologist using a psychoanalytic perspective, believed that lasting psychological damage would be done to a child if the attachment bond between them and their mother was broken by separation. In particular, Bowlby's (1953) theory of maternal deprivation argued that separated children might grow up unable to love or care for others, fail to achieve their educational potential and turn to crime during adolescence and adulthood. Psychologists working outside of the psychoanalytic tradition, such as Michael Rutter (1981), doubted that babies are so seriously affected by separation. Rutter's evidence suggested that it is the quality of the emotional attachment between a baby/child and their carer that matters in promoting psychological development.

See also – Attachment; Loss

References

Bowlby, J. (1953) *Child Care and the Growth of Love*. Harmondsworth: Penguin.
Rutter, M. (1981) *Maternal Deprivation Reassessed*. Harmondsworth: Penguin.

Sexuality

> The concept of sexuality refers to a person's sexual characteristics and sexual behaviour. A person's sexuality incorporates physical, social, psycho-emotional and biological features.

Sexuality is now thought of as being more of a psychosocial issue than a biological one. A person's sexuality doesn't automatically or naturally follow from their biological sex as male or female. In fact, the transgender and non-binary communities (i.e. people who don't identify as either male or female) would dispute that there are only two naturally occurring sexes. Sociologists are interested in patterns of sexuality and sexual behaviour, including the way individuals identify with and form communities based around their sexuality, rather than on the individual psychology of sexuality and sexual orientation. Foucault's (1978) pioneering studies of sexuality moved this area away from biology and into the realm of the social sciences. He did this by exploring histories of sexuality, situating the meaning and experience of sexuality within a historical perspective whilst making visible its connections to social practices, politics and culture.

In its narrowest interpretation, sexuality was closely connected to reproductive processes. This basic, hetero-normative approach presents men and women as naturally attracted to opposite-sex partners and anyone who identifies with a sexuality outside of this as 'abnormal'. Foucault's (1978) studies reveal that until the eighteenth century there was no concept of homosexuality in European societies; distinctions between different forms of sexuality did not carry social or cultural significance until after that time. During the nineteenth century, people attracted to same-sex partners were viewed as aberrant, deviant and a separate type of person. Throughout much of the twentieth century homosexuality was seen as a psychiatric disorder and was socially stigmatised. The decriminalisation of homosexuality in the late twentieth century was part of a cultural shift in attitudes towards sexuality. At the beginning of the twenty-first century,

attitudes towards sexuality are more permissive, even if diverse sexualities are not fully accepted throughout society. Lorber (1994) has identified ten different sexualities including:

- heterosexual woman
- heterosexual man
- lesbian woman
- gay man
- bisexual woman
- bisexual man
- transvestite woman (regularly dressing as a man)
- transvestite man (regularly dressing as a woman)
- transsexual woman (man who becomes a woman)
- transsexual man (woman who becomes a man).

In addition to these diverse sexualities, some people also identify as asexual, claiming they have no sense of sexual desire or sexual attraction towards other people.

Sexuality is an area of social life and experience that social scientists have only recently begun to explore and research. It is an area of life that many people are reluctant to discuss or disclose very much about. However, as society has become more permissive and diversity issues have gained greater recognition, the notion that there are a range of sexualities within the population is now broadly accepted. The social acceptance of a broader range of sexualities has recently led to many countries, including the UK, allowing gay couples to affirm their relationships in legally valid civil partnerships and marriages. Non-heterosexual sexualities, whilst not universally accepted, are no longer discussed and treated as pathological within a medical discourse, although the idea that they are a form of religious 'sin' remains in some faiths.

See also – (The) Body; Identity; Patriarchy

References and further reading

Foucault, M. (1978) *The History of Sexuality*. London, Penguin.

Lorber, J. (1994) *Paradoxes of Gender*. New Haven, CT: Yale University Press.

Richards, C. and Barker, M. (2013) *Sexuality and Gender for Mental Health Professionals*. London: SAGE Publications.

A
B
C
D
E
F
G
H
I
J
K
L
M
N
O
P
Q
R
S
T
U
V
W
X
Y
Z

Sick role

The sick role refers to a set of rights and obligations surrounding illness that shapes the behaviour of doctors and patients in the help-seeking, treatment and recovery process. It is, in essence, a social role that can be occupied by a person who is unwell, that gives them a special status that may have positive and/or negative implications for the person.

Talcott Parsons (1951), an American functionalist sociologist, identified the way in which the sick role played a key part in healthcare practice, experiences and practitioner–patient relationships. Parsons was the first to argue that individuals adopt a socially defined 'sick role' in modern society. He sought to identify how our cultural expectations of what it means to be 'ill' determine how we expect people in this state to behave. Parsons (1951) outlined four components of the 'sick role':

- The sick role legitimately allows social withdrawal and suspension of a person's usual social role obligations – such as going to work or college
- The legitimately sick person is not held to be responsible for their condition
- The sick person is supposed to find the state of being 'sick' undesirable
- The sick role places a social obligation on the sick person to try to get better by using available healthcare resources; therefore, the 'sick' person should not seek to take advantage of the benefits of the sick role (see the first two points).

Doctors play a key part in the sick role through diagnosing illness and then defining an individual as officially 'sick'. Once a person is officially 'sick', they have access to the 'sick role'. A person who does not have a medical diagnosis to legitimise their sickness has to negotiate access to the 'sick role' in other ways and may or may not be successful in doing so. Parsons (1951) argued that the sick role is one way of dealing with ill health in society as it ensures the smooth functioning of society. Its existence, and the need to follow a process of becoming officially 'sick', ensure that the potential disruption that disease and ill health could bring to society is kept to a minimum.

Criticisms of the 'sick role' concept

The concept of the 'sick role' has been criticised for a range of reasons. For example, Parsons (1951) appears to assume that everyone has equal access to the 'sick role'. However, it is clear that, regardless of the problems they face, some people (especially women within families) do not have the option of withdrawing into the sick role. Additionally, there are some occupational and class-based subcultures where adopting the 'sick role' is not viewed positively but rather as a form of personal and moral 'weakness'.

Critics of the concept also argue that it fails to take into account situations where a person is unwilling to adopt or accept the expectations of the 'sick role'. For example, a person who develops epilepsy or a mental disorder, or contracts an infectious disease, may not disclose this because these conditions are socially stigmatised. Additionally, even when the individual who is suffering a particular condition accepts this and seeks to adopt the sick role, their employer, partner or relatives may be reluctant to accept and allow this to happen. For example, a person's relatives may deny the 'reality' of their clinical diagnosis or illness by disputing the medical basis on which it is made. Similarly, it is not uncommon for employers to resist or dispute complaints of 'stress-related illness' that are made by their employees.

Despite these criticisms of the 'sick role' as a concept, it remains a useful way of getting us to think about how society assigns roles and responds to people who claim 'illness'. The moral aspect of 'sick role' judgements is especially important for healthcare providers such as nurses.

See also – Functionalism; Sociological perspective; Stigma

Reference and further reading

Parsons, T. (1951) *The Social System*. Glencoe, IL: Free Press.
White, K. (2017) *An Introduction to the Sociology of Health and Illness*, 3rd edition. London: SAGE Publications.

A
B
C
D
E
F
G
H
I
J
K
L
M
N
O
P
Q
R
S
T
U
V
W
X
Y
Z

Social action and social structure

Structural perspectives, such as functionalism and Marxism, view individuals as relatively powerless to influence their own destiny and life chances. Wider social forces are seen as more important in shaping society than individual social action. By contrast, social action approaches, such as feminist and interactionist perspectives, challenge this assumption. They see social action by individuals and groups who have shared interests (such as women, minority ethnic groups, people with disabilities, etc.) as central to the way in which people are responsible for making and remaking the society they live in.

Social action approaches argue that people create or construct their social experiences through the cultural meanings that they develop and apply in different social situations. Therefore, individual behaviours and the way of life of different groups in society need to be explored and understood in terms of the specific cultural meanings that group members attribute to them. This sociological point is important for healthcare workers who are required to work with a culturally diverse range of people. In a culturally diverse society, a service user's health problems can only be understood by appreciating their cultural perspective and way of life. A healthcare worker who is not culturally sensitive and assumes that everyone views 'health' and 'illness', and experiences life, in the same way will fail to identify why a person has health problems and what can be done (appropriately) to help them overcome them.

Social structure is a sociological concept that refers to the patterned social relationships and practices that both emerge from and determine the actions of individuals.

Sociologists see social structure operating at both a macro or societal level and at a micro or individual, interactional level. At a macro level, social structure is evident in social institutions (such as the family, the education and healthcare systems), in the social class structure and in forms of social stratification based upon social status, gender, ethnicity, disability and age, for example. All of these elements of social life are relatively enduring features of society that have a structuring effect. At a micro level, social norms have a strong but invisible influence on social relations, interaction and behaviour because they become internalised, taken-for-granted 'rules' for social life. As a result, they also have a structuring impact on how social life happens and is experienced.

See also – Functionalism; Marxism; Society; Sociology; Status

Further reading

Haralambos, M. and Holborn, M. (2013) *Sociology Themes and Perspectives*, 8th edition. London: Collins Education.

Social class

> The concept of social class is used to identify a group of people who are similar in terms of their wealth, income and occupation. Social classes are seen to exist in a hierarchical structure in society.

In essence, social classes consist of groups of people who have a similar economic position (type of job, income and status) and often a similar lifestyle, education and shared attitudes and values (see *Table 14*). Social scientists have made widespread use of social class to identify, describe and explain how British society is socially divided and unequal in various ways. A person's social class has been linked to their life chances and health experiences in a large number of social science research studies.

Until 2001, the Registrar-General's scale was used to identify and record an individual's social class position. Statistics based on this scale were developed from census records that held details of the occupation of the male head of each household in Britain. The scale consisted of six social classes

(see *Table 10* in *Mortality and Morbidity*) that were organised into a hierarchy linking occupations to social status.

The influence and significance of social class in contemporary society is an area of continuing debate within the social sciences. It is generally recognised that social class is not as important in the way people define themselves as it used to be in the first half of the twentieth century. However, the UK is far from a 'classless' society – class does still have an impact on an individual's life chances and opportunities. Many social scientists argue that a social class hierarchy does exist within British society and that this has a profound effect on a person's life chances. In particular, there are clear connections between social class and patterns of health and illness experience in society.

Table 14 – The National Statistics Socio-economic classification

Class number	Social class	Types of jobs included
1	Higher managerial and professional occupations	Doctors, lawyers, dentists, professors, professional engineers
2	Lower managerial and professional occupations	School teachers, nurses, journalists, actors, police sergeants
3	Intermediate occupations	Airline cabin crew, secretaries, photographers, firefighters, auxiliary nurses
4	Small employers and own account workers	Self-employed builders, hairdressers, fishing crew, car dealers and shop owners
5	Lower supervisory and technical occupations	Train drivers, employed craftspeople, supervisors
6	Semi-routine occupations	Shop assistants, postal workers, security guards
7	Routine occupations	Bus drivers, waiting staff, cleaners, car park attendants, refuse collectors
8	Never worked or long-term unemployed	Students, people not classifiable, occupations not stated

Social class patterns of mortality

Sociologists have conducted a large number of research studies on the possible effects of social class on life chances. A persistent finding is that a person's social class is the most important predictor of health experience and mortality (death). The key finding that is regularly revealed by sociological data from these studies is that there is a social class gradient in mortality. There is a step-like pattern of increasing mortality from the highest down to the lowest social class. The mortality (death) rate of the lowest social class is approximately twice that of the highest social class. In essence, people in the higher social classes live longer than people in the lower social classes. Richard Wilkinson, a sociological researcher, wrote a letter in 1976 to the social science journal *New Society* about this apparent connection. He asked the Labour government of the time to set up an urgent enquiry into the causes of the link between social class, health experience and death rates. The Black Report of 1980 (Townsend and Davidson, 1988) was the result of the enquiry. This produced hard, empirical evidence of considerable social class differences in health experiences.

The Black Report also showed that differences in death rates between those at the top and those at the bottom of the social class hierarchy had increased during the twentieth century despite the emergence of the National Health Service in the 1940s. For example, in 1930 unskilled workers were 23% more likely to die prematurely than professional workers. By 1970, the likelihood had increased to 61%. The report was very controversial and was initially suppressed by Conservative governments in the 1980s. However, to some sociologists and policy makers this kind of finding provides powerful and compelling evidence of the influence and impact of large-scale structural forces on health and illness experience in British society.

Debates about the social class patterning of health and illness experience have centred on, and often refer back to, the findings of the pioneering Black Report. The report remains significant because it was the first sociological study to provide detailed empirical data showing a social class gradient in health and illness experience. It showed that the lower a person's social class, the more likely they were to experience ill health and to die at an early age. The report showed that in 1980 unskilled workers were still two and a half times more likely to die before retirement than professional workers. More recent data shows that, over the past 20 years, death rates have fallen across all social groups and for both sexes. Despite this, the chances of people from the higher social classes dying early are still falling faster than those of people from lower social classes.

See also – Social action and social structure; Society; Sociology; Status

Reference and further reading

Holborn, M. (2015) *Contemporary Sociology*. Cambridge: Polity Press.

Townsend, P. and Davidson, N. (1988) *Inequalities in Health: the Black Report and the health divide*. Harmondsworth: Penguin.

Social constructionism

Social constructionism is a philosophical approach to knowledge and social reality. It argues that social processes underpin the production of knowledge about the social world. The implication of this is that many aspects of social life that we take for granted and which we assume are 'natural' and real, are, in fact, social constructs.

Social constructionism argues that aspects of contemporary social life and social relations are produced or created (made and remade) through active social processes that have their own histories and which rely on social interaction. For example, the categories of 'race'/ethnicity and sexuality are not neutral or naturally occurring features of human experience. They have been developed and used to make particular sense of human experience at specific times. As such, notions of 'race'/ethnicity and sexuality are not fixed, vary between societies and have changed their meaning over time. In the context of health, illness and the body, social constructionists argue that scientific knowledge – what we currently understand as 'true' – has been produced through subjective, historically determined human interests that are subject to change and reinterpretation. As such, knowledge and ideas about health and illness are never fixed, indisputable or simply 'discovered' through scientific investigation. Instead, social constructionists argue that all knowledge and discourse is created and sustained through social and political processes.

Social constructionism is particularly useful in assessing the way knowledge claims are made within both the natural and social sciences. Paying attention to the historical construction of such claims, identifying and assessing who may benefit and what the ulterior motives for and implications of a knowledge claim might be, tends to open up debate about the claim and issues involved. However, critics of social constructionism argue that it adopts too much of a descriptive, neutral stance on important issues. Exposing and outlining the 'discourse' underpinning a knowledge claim isn't the same thing as engaging with the issue itself.

See also – Interactionism; Realism; Sociological perspective

Further reading

Burr, V. (2015) *Social Constructionism*, 3rd edition. Hove: Routledge.

Social institution

A social institution is an established and enduring pattern of rule-governed behaviour that exists to provide a framework for, or way of dealing with, specific social activities.

In western societies (including the UK) shared 'social' experiences and activities such as raising children, treating illness and disease and developing knowledge and skills occur within 'social institutions'. We call these social institutions 'the family', 'the healthcare system' and 'the education system', respectively. They are contemporary society's way of arranging how best to carry out these shared social tasks. They are also seen as evidence of the existence of a 'society' because they illustrate a collective focus and demonstrate that the human-made world is organised around shared arrangements for meeting collective social needs.

Functionalist sociologists tend to think about and describe 'society' as though it consists of connected social institutions that organise and structure society. These social institutions are often described as the 'building blocks' of society. From this perspective, each of these institutions has a specific role to play in society and must play it effectively for society to work efficiently. The family, the education system, the legal system and health and social care services are all examples of important social institutions that affect the structure of contemporary society. Although each of these institutions is continually developing and changing, they are also relatively permanent features of society. They each have a history of their own, will survive the death of the people who are currently part of them and provide a way of meeting a particular shared need in society.

See also – Families; Functionalism; Social action and social structure; Society

Further reading

Haralambos, M. and Holborn, M. (2013) *Sociology Themes and Perspectives*, 8th edition. London: Collins Education.

Social learning theory

Social learning theory is a psychological perspective that focuses on the influence and impact that relationships and interactions with other people have on human development and behaviour. It is distinctive for the claim that human social behaviour (any behaviour displayed to others) is learned primarily by observing and imitating the actions of others. Social learning theorists argue that behaviour develops because a person is rewarded and/or punished for their actions – or sees others whom they admire being rewarded or punished for specific behaviours.

Bandura and the Bobo Doll experiment

Albert Bandura (b. 1925) is the Canadian psychologist responsible for developing some of the main principles of social learning theory. Bandura recognised that behavioural psychology could only explain how people learn directly through experience. Bandura carried out experiments to show that people, and other animals, also learn *indirectly* by observing and imitating the behaviour of others. As a result, Bandura's social learning theory perspective focuses on the effects that other people, such as parents, teachers, friends, peer group members, celebrities, sports performers and pop stars, for example, can have on an individual's development and behaviour. In particular, Bandura's social learning theory argues that some behaviour is acquired or learnt through imitation of admired people or role models.

Bandura's famous 'Bobo Doll' experiment was used to develop and provide evidence for some of the principles of social learning theory. A Bobo doll is a plastic inflatable toy that stands about 1.5 m tall. It was usually painted with the face of a clown and was bottom-weighted to ensure that if it was hit, it would return to an upright position.

Bandura *et al.*'s (1961) experimental study involved 36 boys and 36 girls, all aged four. In the experiment, the children were divided into three groups (twelve boys and twelve girls in each group) carefully matched for aggression levels. Children were allocated to one of three groups:
1. An aggressive model group, which saw an adult being physically and verbally abusive to a Bobo doll

2. A non-aggressive model group, which saw an adult act neutrally towards a Bobo doll.
3. A third control group, which didn't see an adult playing with the Bobo doll at all.

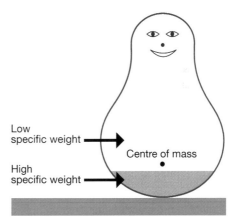

Figure 15 – An example of the type of Bobo doll used in Bandura's experiment.

All of the children spent time in a room with toys they weren't allowed to play with. They were then put in a room with a Bobo doll. Bandura *et al.* (1961) found that the children who were part of the group which saw an adult being verbally and physically aggressive towards the Bobo doll were more likely to treat the doll aggressively themselves than those children who saw the Bobo doll being treated well or who didn't see an adult playing with the doll at all. Bandura's experiment showed that children don't just learn from the consequences of their own actions, but also model the behaviour of others.

Bandura *et al.* (1961) argued that the Bobo doll experiments showed that we learn through a process of imitating role models but that we only imitate behaviour we see as being in our interests. Social learning theorists like Bandura say that for behaviour to be imitated it must be rewarded or reinforced in some way. This can occur through 'vicarious reinforcement' where an individual experiences indirect reinforcement by seeing their role model being reinforced. For example, a child may see their favourite footballer get away with a foul, score a goal and then get lots of praise from team mates and supporters. As a result, they may decide to copy this aspect of their admired role model's behaviour the next time they play football themselves.

The social learning theory approach suggests that learning, and the development of behaviour, sometimes occurs without the need for direct reinforcement. Admired people (role models) are able to influence an individual's behaviour and identity if the individual is motivated to be more like their role model. People are motivated to be more like their role models if they admire or desire the personal attributes or qualities associated with them.

Table 15 – Evaluating social learning theory

What does it offer?	What are its limitations?
Social learning theory combines behaviourist with cognitive principles; this provides a powerful, practical way of promoting learning and behaviour change	Social learning theory does not take into account different levels of ability or an individual's stage of intellectual development – it assumes everyone is capable of learning through observation
The principles of social learning theory are simple, widely used and are seen as effective in educational settings and in care settings where teaching living skills is a feature of care practice	Social learning theory does not take into account the fact that people learn through experimenting and innovating as well as by observing and imitating others – it underplays creativity
The outcomes of a social learning theory approach can be easily observed and are measurable	Social learning theory doesn't explain how to motivate people to learn through imitation – it just suggests that this is what happens and that all people can be motivated in the right circumstances

See also – Classical conditioning; Operant conditioning; Psychological perspective; Reinforcement; Role models

Reference

Bandura, A., Ross, D. and Ross, S.A. (1961) Transmission of aggression through imitation of aggressive models. *Journal of Abnormal and Social Psychology*, **63**: 575–582.

Social mobility

> Social mobility refers to the movement of individuals from one position to another within a society stratified by social class, status, occupation or income group, for example.

Social mobility is typically measured in terms of the economic mobility of individuals and groups in society, using changes in income and wealth (a proxy for social class) as the key indicators of social mobility. A person may experience upward or downward social mobility. An individual or group that has seen a relative increase or decrease in their income or wealth over time is likely to have experienced social mobility – they have moved up or down the socio-economic scale or ladder in society. A second way of identifying social mobility is to focus on occupation. Again, social scientists measure the social mobility of individuals and groups by comparing their occupational status at a particular point in their lives with that of their parents (usually their father). Social mobility may be reported as intergenerational (between one or more generations) or intragenerational (within the same generation). Intergenerational mobility is more frequently cited and used by social scientists when exploring or discussing social mobility issues.

Sociologists argue that social mobility is an important concept because it provides a measure of the openness, fluidity and structural features of society. The concept of social mobility also appears in political debates about fairness, equality of opportunity and access to power in society. There has been considerable research, discussion and debate in social science to try to identify the key factors that trigger social mobility and which explain why it is or isn't happening during a particular period of time. Power, the reproduction of social class advantages and access to education have all been seen as important influences in this respect. Pierre Bourdieu's (1977) concept of different types of 'capital' has also provided a way of understanding the drivers of social mobility in society.

Bourdieu argued that three types of capital place a person in a certain social category. These are: economic capital, social capital and cultural capital. Economic capital refers to the economic resources available to a person or group in society (cash, credit and other material assets). Social capital refers to the resources that result from membership of different social groups, networks of influence and relationships to other people. Cultural capital refers to the status advantages that a person obtains through acquiring education, skills and other forms of valued knowledge. People with all three types of capital tend to be in a higher status, more advantaged position in society. In this way, the acquisition, or loss, of economic, social or cultural capital can be linked to the experience of social mobility.

Social scientists, politicians and economists tend to agree that some social mobility is good for society and that low, or no, social mobility is likely to have negative consequences. Efforts to compare social mobility across societies are difficult because societies and their economies may not be similar enough to allow direct comparison. As such, there is no international measure of social mobility. It is possible, however, to use longitudinal data, such as child development and economic data, to compare how much social mobility is achieved by cohorts of people born at different times within a society. Analysis of those data sets can reveal trends in patterns of intragenerational social mobility.

See also –Social action and social structure; Social class; Status

Reference and further reading

Bourdieu, P. (1977) 'Cultural Reproduction and Social Reproduction' in J. Karabel and A.H. Halsey (eds) *Power and Ideology in Education*. Oxford: Oxford University Press.

Social model of health

The social model of health is an approach to understanding and explaining health and illness experience that prioritises the role of social and psychological factors and which proposes that social change, social support and psychological interventions can improve health outcomes for individuals, within communities and at a whole population level.

The social model of health is often seen as an alternative to the orthodox and dominant biomedical approach. It shouldn't be seen as a rejection of biomedicine although it is often drawn on in critiques of biomedicine. Biomedical knowledge and medical practitioners have an important role to play in healthcare provision. Medicine has a very important role to play in 'fighting' disease and 'saving lives', for example, but there are plenty of arguments and sources of evidence to show that biomedicine is useful only for some of the 'health' problems that people face, rather than for everything. Sociologists have noted that the growth of interest in complementary therapies and public health has led to a shift towards social models of health and illness, and new, community-based approaches to the provision of services.

During the nineteenth century, the tradition of public health medicine developed alongside, but separate from, the biological/individual focus of the biomedical model. Both shared a negative definition of health as being the absence of illness. However, the public health model attempted, through preventive methods such as improving water supplies, and developing public housing programmes and health education campaigns, to prevent general ill health from occurring in society in the first place.

The public health approach adopts a socio-medical model of health. The real causes and origins of ill health are seen as being located in the environment rather than the individual. For example, poor housing and poverty are environmental factors that contribute to respiratory problems. The 'public health' solution is better housing and programmes to tackle inequality and poverty. The medical model solution consists of antibiotics to treat the pathology, or malfunctioning, that is occurring in the individual's respiratory system.

See also – Anti-psychiatry; Biomedical model; Discourse; Science

Further reading

Tew, J. (2011) *Social Approaches to Mental Distress*. Basingstoke: Palgrave.
White, K. (2017) *An Introduction to the Sociology of Health and Illness*, 3rd edition. London: SAGE Publications.

Social policy

The key focus of social policy in the UK is on social welfare provision. Social policy is essentially concerned with the practice and study of state, or governmental, social welfare provision, and the healthcare and welfare systems. People who study British social policy focus on why, what and how social welfare is provided by British governments.

Social policy as a subject has its roots in the social sciences, and is relevant to students who have an interest in the provision of 'social welfare' and the operation of health and welfare services. It is now widely studied as a subject in itself, and is also increasingly likely to be a part of social science and health and social care courses. These kinds of courses cover key 'social welfare' issues such as health, poverty and education.

Social policy is particularly concerned with:
- ideologies, values and beliefs about individuals, society and 'social welfare'
- real-world, contemporary 'social problems'
- the approaches and actions of governments and the state to 'social welfare' issues
- the political, social and economic context of social policy-making and its implementation
- the nature and effectiveness of health and social welfare provision in the UK.

Social policy has a major impact on the goals, focus and everyday work of health and social care organisations and practitioners who work within them.

See also – Community; Socialism; Welfare; Welfare state

Further reading

Alcock, P. and May, M. (2014) *Social Policy in Britain*, 4th edition. Basingstoke: Palgrave Macmillan.

Sealey, C. (2015) *Social Policy Simplified: connecting theory and concepts with people's lives.* Basingstoke: Palgrave Macmillan.

Social support

The concept of 'support' is generally understood to be a psychosocial feature of relationships. People give and receive support within relationships and also have a felt, or subjective, sense of whether their relationship(s) with another person is supportive. The support that people offer to, and receive from, each other can be emotional (e.g. nurturance), tangible (e.g. financial assistance), informational (e.g. advice), based on companionship (e.g. a sense of belonging) or more intangible (e.g. personal connection). All of the different forms of support can be experienced as helpful, depending on the person's needs and how they are offered or provided.

Health and social care workers are encouraged to develop and maintain supportive relationships with patients/service users. Part of the reason for this is that being supportive keeps the person engaged and involved in the relationship, but it also contributes to their health and wellbeing. Leach (2015), for example, suggests social support has beneficial effects on mental health and wellbeing. He describes the social support that people provide for each other as "the everyday help and reassurance that friends, relatives, colleagues and others give each other throughout their lives. It can both protect against mental distress and help people cope with the effects of mental health problems".

When support is contrasted with 'care' it is usually seen as being less structured, deliberate or technical (e.g. social support vs. medical care). It tends to be seen as a relationship-based form of assistance typically provided by non-professionals. For example, when a care practitioner is assessing whether a person has sufficient 'social support' they are thinking about whether there is a network of friends, family and acquaintances (such as neighbours and work colleagues) surrounding the person. This kind of informal social support is important for both physical and mental health because a lack of social support is associated with social isolation and feelings of loneliness. Even when a person has a social network they can still feel lonely if those relationships are unsupportive or actually detrimental to their wellbeing. Social support is not just a matter of how many people you know but of how supportive you find your relationship(s) with them.

Social scientists and health and social care practitioners became more interested in the role of social support in society, and its impact on health and wellbeing, in the 1980s. Clarifying both the nature of social support and its benefits, Albrecht and Adelman (1987) argued that there are three main aspects to social support interactions:

- They meet a need for human contact, which involves making sense of one's life and the events that occur within it.
- Supportive interactions help reduce feelings of uncertainty, both about the situation a person finds themselves in and about their relationship with the other person. This leads to the person having a greater sense of control over their life and over the stressful conditions that might adversely affect them.
- Social support takes place within a structure of connected and reciprocal relationships, some strong, some weak, in which help is given and received.

Turner and Brown (2010) have since referred to social support as a multidimensional construct comprising:

- perceived support – knowing support is available if needed
- structural support – the presence of social ties and a network that can be used as a resource
- received support – the actual provision of helpful information or practical assistance provided by others.

Health and social care practitioners now recognise that social support helps people to feel (and be) connected with each other, gives people a valued identity and enables people to deal with stressful conditions more effectively. In addition to assessing the extent to which a person has social support available to them, care practitioners will often develop care and treatment plans based around the provision of social support and which aim to introduce, develop or extend the social support a person has available to them.

There are many ways of doing this but at the heart of all of them is connecting a person to others through positive, nurturing relationships.

See also – Biomedical model; Social model of health; Welfare

References

Albrecht, T.L. and Adelman, M. (1987) *Communicating Social Support*. London: SAGE Publications.

Leach, J. (2015) *Improving Mental Health Through Social Support: building positive and empowering relationships*. London: Jessica Kingsley Publishers.

Turner, R. and Brown, R. (2010) 'Social support and mental health', in T. Scheid and T. Brown (eds) *A Handbook for the Study of Mental Health: social contexts, theories and systems*. New York: Cambridge University Press.

A
B
C
D
E
F
G
H
I
J
K
L
M
N
O
P
Q
R
S
T
U
V
W
X
Y
Z

Socialisation

Socialisation is the process through which individuals acquire and internalise the norms, values and culture of their society and learn how to express these in socially acceptable behaviour.

Socialisation refers to the process through which individuals learn the roles, norms and culture of a social group or society. Primary socialisation occurs in the family during a child's early years. Children learn (or 'catch') social attitudes, values and acceptable ways of behaving from observing, and being informally educated by, parents, siblings and other significant relatives. However, sociologists also recognise that socialisation is a lifelong process. It continues during adolescence and adulthood into middle and old age. Secondary socialisation occurs outside of the family. Friends and peers, school mates, work colleagues, the media, role models, religious leaders and influential people such as teachers and employers are all agents of secondary socialisation.

How does socialisation affect us?

Sociologists argue that it is through socialisation processes that we all learn how to become members of society and develop a sense of self. Socialisation is the social science concept that explains how human beings change from biological entities into social beings. We are born without any sense or knowledge of culture or of the values or norms of society. Culture, values and norms are transmitted to us though primary socialisation and then secondary socialisation. This enables us to relate to, fit in with and understand other members of society. Socialisation also plays a key part in forming an individual's personal and social identities. Many aspects of identity are formed through our particular experiences of family, friends, school, the mass media and the workplace, for example. We are affected by the way others see us and the way we define ourselves in these contexts, identifying with some groups or institutions and not others. In this way our sense of 'who' we are (our 'self') is shaped by, and is also a response to, lots of socialisation influences. Consequently, we learn how to perform certain social roles – as brother/sister, student, employee, for example – and also acquire and take into account the status of these roles when relating to others.

See also – Culture; Social institution; Social learning theory; Society

Further reading

Haralambos, M. and Holborn, M. (2013) *Sociology Themes and Perspectives*, 8th edition. London: Collins Education.

Socialism

Socialism is a political ideology and approach to economic organisation that proposes collective ownership and government control of major industries and public services, rather than private ownership and control by individuals and companies in a free market.

Socialism's focus on collective ownership and government control of the economy and public services aims to address the socio-economic inequalities that are apparent in capitalist societies. Socialism developed and grew as a response to the inequalities that emerged following the Industrial Revolution when private ownership of the means of production led to pronounced inequalities in wealth and in living standards between owners of land and businesses and the much larger number of agricultural and industrial workers. Socialists tend to argue that collective or shared ownership of the means of production and government provision of public services ensure a level of social equality or fairness that is lacking in an exploitative and inequitable capitalist system. Socialism claims to offer an equitable distribution of resources, equality of opportunity for all and greater democracy because it focuses on the common good.

See also – Capitalism; Social policy; Welfare state

Further reading

Alcock, P. and May, M. (2014) *Social Policy in Britain*, 4th edition. Basingstoke: Palgrave Macmillan.
Newman, M. (2005) *Socialism: a very short introduction*. Oxford: Oxford University Press.

Society

Society is a set of social institutions and patterns of social relations that connect a large community of people.

One of the fundamental tenets of sociology is that people bound together in a collective enterprise live in 'societies'. The term 'society' has a variety of meanings but is typically used to identify the general collectivity to which we belong and which is more than the sum of its parts. 'Societies' are also seen to involve networks of people relating to each other in meaningful ways.

Sociologists began using the term 'society' in the way we now understand it in the nineteenth century. In many ways it is a fundamental concept of sociology. In fact, many definitions of the subject define it as 'the study of societies'. It focuses us on the collective experience of human life, distinguishing sociology's broader, outward-looking whole society focus from the individual level, inward-looking focus of psychology. From its earliest uses, the concept of 'society' has typically been associated with a collectivity living in a bounded, geographical territory. In particular, a 'society' seemed to assume the existence and boundaries of a nation state. As a result, sociologists have consistently compared and contrasted particular societies and their structures and processes (e.g. industrial vs. pre-industrial societies). They have also focused on issues such as inequalities and power relations within national societies, as well as how processes of social change have shifted societies from one stage or type to another (e.g. industrial to post-industrial, feudal to capitalist, modern to postmodern societies).

The continuing usefulness of the concept of 'society' has been questioned and criticised from within and outside of sociology since the 1970s. In particular the association between 'society' and the nation state makes it seem like a static idea and presents 'society' as a 'thing' existing outside of the activities and social practices of the individuals who are part of it. Sociologists critical of this approach have put forward the argument that society is made and remade through and within the social relations and interactions that occur between individuals and communities and question how 'society' can exist outside of social relations. Additionally, globalisation now challenges the notion of the geographically bounded society. People, goods and services are constantly moving across national boundaries whilst personal, political, commercial and cultural relationships often span borders without being thought of as being cross-societal. Multinational corporations (Google, Microsoft and Amazon, for example) and supranational organisations (e.g. European Union, World Bank, United Nations) are often wealthier and more powerful than individual countries or nations. These organisations operate above and have a level of social influence beyond that of a nation/society and are arguably becoming more effective in shaping social life. The globalisation thesis suggests that the concept of a coexisting nation/society is, in fact, rapidly becoming redundant as global mobilities and flows of goods, services and people move us all towards a 'global society'.

See also – Globalisation; Social institution

Further reading

Haralambos, M. and Holborn, M. (2013) *Sociology Themes and Perspectives*, 8th edition. London: Collins Education.

Wilkinson, I. and Kleinman, A. (2016) *A Passion for Society: how we think about human suffering*. Oakland, CA: University of California Press.

Sociological perspective

> A sociological perspective is a theoretical way of analysing, understanding and explaining society, social practices and social relations.

There are a variety of different, sometimes competing, ways of looking at the structure and processes of the social world. These can be categorised in the following ways.

- *Structural perspectives*, such as functionalism and Marxism, that see social structures and institutions as being the main factors shaping 'society' and influencing our social experiences. Functionalism views society as composed of different, interconnected parts working together to achieve social stability. In contrast, Marxism is a conflict perspective that views society as composed of different class-based groups with antagonistic interests competing for power and resources.
- *Social action or interpretivist perspectives*, such as symbolic interactionism and ethnomethodology, focus on the micro-level social relationships and psychological dynamics that occur when individuals form and interact in small groups and communities. Social action approaches see society as being made and remade at the micro-level where meaning, identity and our sense of self are shaped by social interaction.
- *Standpoint perspectives*, such as feminism, anti-racism and environmentalism.
- Postmodern perspectives.

Each perspective provides a distinct way of understanding and explaining the social world. Sociologists tend to suggest, usually implicitly, that the perspective informing their research or theoretical approach is the best way of gaining a clear, insightful understanding of the aspect of the social world they're focusing on. As a result, sociologists using other perspectives tend to contest or argue about the validity and usefulness of each other's claims. As a result, arguments about how the social world really works or can be best understood are an ongoing feature of sociological debate.

Students new to social science tend to develop an affinity or liking for one or more perspectives at the expense of others. However, it is advisable to avoid becoming blindly committed to one perspective on the basis that it *really* does offer an answer to every sociological issue or problem. This is never the case. Instead it is worth exploring what insights each perspective can offer when it is used to analyse particular issues or social phenomena. Different perspectives tend to focus on and offer useful insights into different features of the social world in the same way that different keys open different doors.

See also – Functionalism; Interactionism; Marxism; Social action and social structure

Further reading

Haralambos, M. and Holborn, M. (2013) *Sociology Themes and Perspectives*, 8th edition. London: Collins Education.

Sociology

The term 'sociology' has Latin and Greek origins and means 'reasoning about the social'. Auguste Comte (1798–1857), a French philosopher who lived through the turbulent social upheavals of the French Revolution of 1789 and the subsequent counter-revolutions, is often given credit for coining the term 'sociology'.

The early nineteenth century period, in which 'sociology' emerged, was an era of massive social change. The French Revolution and the longer Industrial Revolution were responsible for reshaping the institutions and 'fabric' of European societies. Social and political relationships were redefined during this period as the power of the Church, the monarchy and the wealthy landed aristocracy was diminished in the face of challenges from utopian social reformers and political revolutionaries. Comte's 'sociology' was an attempt to understand the social changes that were occurring in France during this period and also a grander effort to develop a 'science of society' that could be used to promote progressive social change in the future.

The pioneers of sociology, such as Auguste Comte, established some of the key themes of sociology that remain a part of the discipline today. For example, since the early nineteenth century sociology has focused on:

- discovering, and describing the effects of, the dynamics of social change
- identifying and describing social structures and processes
- explaining the relationship between the individual and collective 'society'.

The discipline of sociology has evolved and increased in popularity over the last 200 years. It gained greater coherence and much of its academic credibility in the last half of the twentieth century. At the beginning of the twenty-first century, sociology is an established and widely studied academic discipline in its own right. It has a global presence in educational and training institutions, for example, and has generated a substantial body of theoretical and research-based literature on all kinds of specialist sociological topics. As you are now becoming aware, applying sociological theories and methods to areas such as healthcare has put the subject on the timetables of many different professional training courses. The courses, like your own, in which sociology now features, are typically preparing students for 'human services' roles or have a close interest in what has been referred to as 'the human-made world' (Bauman and May, 2001). It is these aspects of the world, the bits that "bear the imprint of human activity, that would not exist at all but for the actions of human beings" (Bauman and May, 2001), that sociology as a subject is concerned with.

Sociology and other healthcare subjects

Pre-qualifying training courses for healthcare practitioners, including nurses, usually cover a range of foundation subject areas. These tend to include the so-called 'natural sciences' (biology, biochemistry, anatomy and physiology, for example) and the 'social sciences' as well as clinical practice and skills inputs. As a result, pre-qualifying courses adopt something of a 'magpie approach' to their knowledge base. They take or borrow theories, concepts and research approaches from the subject areas that are most useful for developing an understanding of the health field.

Sociology is often identified as a 'social science' discipline within this 'pick and mix' selection. There is a significant debate within and outside of sociology circles about whether it is, or should even seek to be, a 'scientific' discipline. However, despite this, sociology is usually categorised alongside psychology, social policy, anthropology, politics and economics as a 'social' science discipline because, like these other subjects, sociology focuses on human activity and experience. Sociology and psychology are the two social science subjects that are most often drawn on in healthcare training courses.

If the social sciences are a new area of study for you, the distinctions between psychology and sociology may be difficult to work out at first. This problem partly occurs because psychology and sociology do 'overlap' at times. It's true that sociologists and psychologists are often interested in exploring similar (sometimes the same) 'human world' topics and issues. However, it's important to note that if sociologists and psychologists do explore the same aspects of the human world they are likely to do so using differing theoretical approaches and by employing research methods in distinctive ways.

What is different about sociology?

A simple way of distinguishing between psychology and sociology is to say that psychology typically focuses on internal aspects of *the individual*. Psychologists generally investigate and develop theories about the factors and processes that affect our internal psychological and emotional processes and behaviours. They're interested in 'personality', 'emotions', 'learning', 'memory' and 'thinking', for example. The individual is, therefore, the main object or focus of psychological research. In contrast, sociology focuses on how aspects of 'the human world' which are external to people affect us *as a collective*. It is more concerned with how external 'social' and 'environmental' factors and processes work together. These are seen to construct and coordinate the life chances and experiences of human beings *at a group level* (as, for example, 'nurses', 'pregnant women', 'African–Caribbean men') and within the context of society as a whole. Sociologists are, therefore, interested in 'social class', 'ethnicity' and 'gender' as fields of social relations within the 'human-made world' that affect people at a collective, or group, level.

Sociology is sometimes seen as being concerned with major social problems, such as unemployment, poverty and racism, which affect some people's lives. These aspects of the human world are important and interesting to some people in the sociology community. However, identifying and addressing social problems and the welfare needs of people who experience them is typically the focus of another discipline – social policy. Sociology is one of several disciplines that social policy academics and practitioners draw on. In particular, social policy practitioners are likely to use sociological thinking and research methods to investigate how and why aspects of the contemporary human world, such as 'social structures', 'social relationships' and 'socio-economic processes', may create the conditions in which these social problems can occur.

See also – Social policy; Society; Sociological perspective

Reference and further reading

Bauman, Z. and May, T. (2001) *Thinking Sociologically*, 2nd edition. Oxford: Blackwell Publishers.
Haralambos, M. and Holborn, M. (2013) *Sociology Themes and Perspectives*, 8th edition. London: Collins Education.

Status

Within social science, the concept of status refers to the rank or position of a person or group within society or a social group. In addition to identifying position within a social system, the concept of status is also used as a measure of prestige or social standing. A person's position can carry positive or negative status within a social system. It may be significant for them, in terms of influencing their sense of identity and access to opportunities and to others who take it into account when relating or responding to them on the basis of their apparent status.

Social scientists distinguish between achieved status (such as through passing exams and gaining qualifications) and ascribed status (obtained via inheritance or appointment). Sociologists also refer to embodied status which is generated through physical characteristics such as visible disability, physical stature/build, skin colour, sex or beauty, for example. These different forms and uses of 'status' are significant in everyday life because the relative rank or status a person has with a society or social hierarchy group is closely linked to their rights, duties, opportunities and lifestyle, for example.

Status is often indicated by occupation in modern societies. Membership of other social groups, such as gender, class and age groupings, is also influential and links this concept to that of intersectionality. However, status is most closely linked to class, wealth (e.g. socio-economic status) and access to power in society. In this sense people with higher status, i.e. a higher social ranking, in their workplace, community or society in general, tend to have better incomes, more wealth and greater control over the work or other activities of people beneath them in the social ranking. Social scientists tend to argue that all societies have a status hierarchy.

Status is relevant to nursing practice where hospitals and other healthcare settings operate on the basis of a hierarchical set of prescribed roles, each accorded an accountability and level of authority that gives the person occupying the role a particular status. For example, staff nurses are accountable to ward sisters or ward manager who are accountable to modern matrons in a typical occupational status hierarchy in nursing. In theory, higher status is given on the basis of experience, higher qualifications and expertise. This may not be the case in practice, although higher status does tend to be reflected in better salaries.

See also – Authority; Identity; Intersectionality; Social class

Further reading

Marmot, M. (2015) *Status Syndrome: how your place on the social gradient directly affects your health*. London: Bloomsbury.

Stereotyping

Social scientists use the term stereotyping to describe the way in which a person or group of people can be categorised or defined in a limited or limiting way.

Stereotypes tend to be based on biased or at least partial assumptions about an individual or group. They could focus on physical appearance or characteristics, or on social attributes or roles. Social scientists have identified the way a range of social factors can lead people and groups to be stereotyped. These include sex, age, physical disability, class, nationality, ethnicity, sexual orientation and mental status, for example.

Stereotypes are not objective or neutral classifications of 'types of people'. Social scientists argue that stereotypes are developed, informed and maintained by political, social and cultural value systems and are used by dominant groups and social institutions to maintain and justify privilege and power over more disadvantaged groups in society.

Health and social care workers often work with individuals and groups who have been unfairly stereotyped (e.g. people experiencing mental illness, disabled people, lone parents) and who are perceived, judged and treated in terms of a dominant stereotype of 'who' and what kind of people they are. Part of their professional role is to resist and counter the effects of negative stereotyping, to ensure that each person is treated fairly and equally as an individual rather than in stereotypical terms. Stereotyping involves disempowering and depersonalising the individual or group in ways that can deny their right to self-determination, self-expression and respect from others.

See also – Attitudes; Discrimination; Prejudice

Further reading

Dovidio, J., Hewstone, M., Glick, P. and Esses, V.M. (2010) *The SAGE Handbook of Prejudice, Stereotyping and Discrimination*. London: SAGE Publications.

Stigma

Social stigma is a concept that refers to the discrediting, devaluation or 'spoiling' of a person's social identity. Essentially, people who suffer some form of social stigma acquire an 'undesired differentness' that taints and reduces them in the eyes of others. Researchers using labelling theory have outlined how social stigma has a significant impact on the lives of those who are diagnosed (i.e. labelled) as 'epileptic' (Scambler and Hopkins, 1986; Scambler, 1989), with HIV/AIDS (Alonzo and Reynolds, 1995; Lawless *et al.*, 1996) and suffering from 'mental illness' (Link and Cullen, 1983).

People who acquire, or are at risk of acquiring, an illness diagnosis that is stigmatised can find the social stigma more difficult to cope with than the condition itself. Sociologists have developed a number of explanations of how people react to, and try to cope with, the social stigma associated with stigmatising illness labels. For example, Erving Goffman (1963) distinguished between conditions, illnesses or impairments that are *discrediting* and those that are *discreditable*. Where a person's stigmatised condition, illness or impairment is visible and affects their social interaction with others, Goffman argued that it acts as a discrediting attribute. People can see that the person is different in some way and, acting according to dominant beliefs and values, react negatively towards this culturally defined 'abnormality'. In response, people with discrediting attributes often try to use 'impression management' strategies. These seek to avoid, challenge and/or overcome the negative stereotypes and devalued identities that are associated with particular 'illness' labels.

Goffman suggests that, where a person's condition, illness or impairment is invisible, they have the option of trying to keep it a secret. Because 'hidden' or invisible illness labels are only potentially discrediting, the main challenge for people who are subject to them is one of 'information management'.

Scambler and Hopkins (1986) carried out a study of the reactions of people to a diagnosis of 'epilepsy'. Extending Goffman's work on the strategies open to people with stigmatising conditions, they explored and theorised about the personal impact that the diagnosis had on people living with this label. They proposed that,

while people often challenged the socially stigmatising label of 'epileptic', they still experienced 'hidden distress'. Scambler and Hopkins (1986) argued that 'hidden distress' results from a fear of *enacted stigma* and a sense of *felt stigma*. Enacted stigma occurs where a person publicly experiences prejudice and discrimination because of their 'epilepsy'/'epileptic' labels. Felt stigma occurs where the person experiences the social shame of being labelled 'epileptic' and also fears the occurrence of enacted stigma should their diagnosis be revealed to others. As a result their social identity, behaviour and view of the world are shaped and coloured by the effects (actual and potential) of social stigma.

In a study of people diagnosed with HIV, Alonzo and Reynolds (1995) proposed that participants also experienced a 'stigma trajectory' alongside their 'illness trajectory'. That is, the nature and degree of stigma attributed to, and experienced by, people who are HIV positive changes over the course of the illness. Alonzo and Reynolds (1995) outlined four phases of the stigma trajectory:

1. **At risk**: this occurs prior to diagnosis and is characterised by uncertainty. The possibility of an HIV-positive diagnosis causes people to experience a 'potentially felt stigma'. There are a variety of responses to this, including denial and the rejection of 'risk'.
2. **Diagnostic**: 'information management' is the key issue at this stage. Who should be told about the stigmatised diagnosis? 'Felt stigma' is likely to occur here.
3. **Latent**: the individual can conceal their diagnosis and illness condition for a certain amount of time while asymptomatic. Felt stigma is likely, but

enacted stigma can be avoided during this phase of the illness and stigma trajectories.

4. **Manifest**: 'deviant' status can no longer be concealed when signs and symptoms of the person's HIV illness become obvious. The person is now more likely to experience enacted stigma at this point in their illness trajectory.

Alonzo and Reynolds' (1995) conceptualisation of the 'stigma trajectory' is useful for showing how the impact of social stigma can vary during a person's illness experience.

See also – Anti-psychiatry; Attitudes; Discrimination; Identity; Labelling; Prejudice

References

Alonzo, A.A. and Reynolds, N.R. (1995) Stigma, HIV and AIDS: an exploration and elaboration of a stigma trajectory. *Social Science and Medicine*, **41:** 303–315.

Goffman, E. (1963) *Stigma: notes on the management of spoiled identity.* Englewood Cliffs, NJ: Prentice-Hall.

Lawless, S., Kippax, S. and Crawford, J. (1996) Dirty, diseased and undeserving: the position of HIV positive women. *Social Science and Medicine*, 43: 1371–1377.

Link, B.G. and Cullen, F.T. (1983) Reconsidering the social rejection of ex-mental patients: levels of attitudinal response. *American Journal of Community Psychology*, **11:** 261–273.

Scambler, G. (1989) *Epilepsy.* London: Routledge.

Scambler, G. and Hopkins, A. (1986) Being epileptic: coming to terms with stigma. *Sociology of Health and Illness*, 8: 26–43.

Stress (and coping)

In psychology, stress is a feeling of strain and pressure when faced by difficult or demanding challenges.

Small amounts of stress may be desired, beneficial, and even healthy. In fact, positive stress ('eustress') helps improve athletic and work performance. It also plays a factor in motivation, adaptation, and reaction to the environment. However, health and social care workers tend to focus on the state of psychological tension caused by excessive stress ('distress') that has a negative effect on people, making them feel they are unable to cope with everyday living and work demands.

The notion that a person's lifestyle, work situation or personal life can have a stressful effect on them is widely held. In some situations, stress may be the consequence of personal decisions and choices. For example, some people choose to do work that is personally challenging or to work long hours to make more money. Alternatively, a combination of unavoidable factors – poor housing, debts, loss of employment, relationship breakdown, health problems – may result in a person developing a stress-related condition.

Stress can affect people in a variety of ways. Research suggests that stress experienced in infancy and childhood can have a significant effect on social and emotional development throughout life. For example, fear and uncertainty undermine the development of confidence and self-esteem. Additionally, children and adolescents who are more stressed are less likely to learn well or realise their intellectual potential. High levels of stress in adulthood and old age can disrupt and damage a person's social relationships and have a negative effect on their self-esteem and confidence. Extreme, sudden stress as well as more low level, continuous or chronic stress is linked to a range of physical health problems, including depression, anxiety, eczema, asthma, high blood pressure, heart disease and stomach ulcers. Stress reduces the quality of a person's life, has a negative effect on their development and will probably lead to physical and mental health problems unless it is reduced or dealt with.

See also – Anxiety; Cognitive behavioural therapy; Defence mechanisms; Dissonance; Mental illness; Mortality and Morbidity

Further reading

Cromby, J., Harper, D. and Reavey, P. (2013) *Psychology, Mental Health and Distress.* Basingstoke: Palgrave Macmillan.

Gross, R. (2015) *Psychology: the science of mind and behaviour*, 7th edition. London: Hodder Education.

Unconscious mind

The unconscious mind is a concept associated with psychoanalysis and psychodynamic or 'deep' psychology.

Sigmund Freud (1856–1939), the founding father of psychoanalysis, developed a revolutionary and influential psychological theory to explain the human mind and behaviour. Part of this argued that human behaviour and thinking can be motivated by 'unconscious' processes.

Freud believed that the mind consisted of three territories. These are the conscious, the pre-conscious and the unconscious parts of the mind. The conscious mind is aware of the here and now, functioning when the person is awake so that the person behaves in a rational, thoughtful way. For example, right now your conscious mind includes the words you are reading. This level or part of the mind handles all the information you receive from the outside world through your senses. The pre-conscious mind lies just below the surface of consciousness and contains partially forgotten ideas and feelings. It can be compared to a filing cabinet where we store everything we need to remember and which we can bring to conscious awareness easily. It also prevents disturbing unconscious memories from surfacing. The unconscious mind is the biggest part and acts as a store of all the memories, feelings and ideas that the individual experiences throughout life. The things that lurk deep in the unconscious are seen to play a powerful, ongoing role in influencing the person's emotions, behaviour and personality.

Freud claimed that the development and expression of a person's emotions and behaviour are driven by three interrelated structures – the Id, Ego and Super-ego. According to Freud, the Id and Super-ego are always in conflict. The Id, or unconscious part of the personality, is focused on getting what it wants. It consists of sexual, aggressive and loving instincts and wants immediate gratification. The Super-ego is the last part of the personality to develop as a result of socialisation. Morals and a sense of right and wrong drive it – it is the person's 'conscience'. The Ego tries to balance the demands of the Id and Super-ego. It is the conscious, rational part of the personality.

See also – Freud; Psychoanalysis; Psychodynamic perspective

Further reading

Gross, R. (2015) *Psychology: the science of mind and behaviour*, 7th edition. London: Hodder Education.

Underclass

The controversial concept of an underclass developed from a conservative political analysis of the social class structure in American society. The 'underclass' is seen as the section of the population at the very bottom of the class hierarchy. It sits beneath the working class and is viewed as being dependent on welfare benefits, engaged in low-level criminal activity and prone to poor lifestyle choices and child-rearing judgements.

The existence and definition of the 'underclass' has been widely and hotly debated in the social sciences. The concept was popularised by Charles Murray in a book about the American welfare system, *Losing Ground* (1983/2015). His argument, since extended to Britain, is that welfare systems create dependency and trap people in poverty and a workless lifestyle. Social scientists have disputed both the data Murray used and the conclusions that he came to. However, the arguments that he made, linking a particular group of people to a psychologically deviant mindset of beliefs, opinions and material desires that reject education and conventional means of work-based achievement in favour of welfare dependency, petty criminality and poor moral choices, has resonated with some right-wing political views.

Social scientists tend to reject the idea that there is an identifiable group of people in an underclass position. However, the term is used in discussions and debates about social inequality and social exclusion. In particular, there is concern that those in the poorest social groups are at risk of becoming mentally and materially disconnected from society, develop beliefs and feelings that they are outside of society and feel that they cannot participate and achieve what they want through legitimate means. Critics of the concept feel that it has been used by right-wing governments to develop education, welfare and social policies to blame those experiencing poverty, unemployment, crime and welfare dependency for their own problems. The argument is that this conflates a number of social problems into a victim-blaming approach that points to a 'culture of poverty' and a subculture that marginalises itself.

See also – Inequalities; Social action and social structure; Social class

Reference and further reading

Murray, C. (1983/2015) *Losing Ground: American social policy 1950–1980*. New York: BasicBooks.

Welshman, J. (2013) *Underclass: a history of the excluded since 1880*, 2nd edition. London: Bloomsbury Academic.

Urbanisation

Urbanisation refers to the movement of populations from rural to urban areas.

The eighteenth and nineteenth centuries saw a major shift in the location of the British population from rural to urban areas. The growth of factories in new conurbations and the availability of work in them initially attracted people away from the countryside and then sustained higher densities of people in urban areas. This process of urbanisation is a global phenomenon. It is estimated that half of the world's population lived in urban areas by the end of 2008. The United Nations has also predicted that by 2050 64% of the developing world and 86% of the developed world will be urbanised. The majority of global population growth is now absorbed by cities.

Sociologists, public health specialists and economists are all interested in the process and impact of urbanisation on society. Urbanisation is sometimes viewed as a process that impacts an area or country within a set time period. More broadly, the impact and implications of urbanisation on housing, employment and health and wellbeing have been studied over extended time periods. The demand for, allocation and use of resources and their impact on social life in urbanised environments, as well as the impact of these processes on the natural environment, have been the focus of considerable research effort. Mass migration and the continuing growth of urbanised, city environments have a major impact on the physical and social conditions in which people live. The consequences of a mass of people being drawn to an already densely populated area can include:

- housing shortages and squalor
- sanitation and public health problems
- fewer work opportunities and exploitation of workers.

Social scientists who are interested in the impact that urbanisation can have on issues such as health and wellbeing often compare the experiences of people in urbanised settings to those living in rural settings. Lifestyles, social networks and employment opportunities as well as access to and experiences of healthcare services can be significantly different in each type of setting. This can mean that health problems can be overlooked, or hidden in less populated rural areas and that health and other support services can be less well resourced and less accessible. It is not unusual, for example, for rurally-based services to be 'relocated' to a more urban setting as part of an organisation's efficiency and rationalisation strategy.

See also – Industrialisation; Social policy

Further reading

Haralambos, M. and Holborn, M. (2013) *Sociology Themes and Perspectives*, 8th edition. London: Collins Education.

Values

Values are moral values or principles that inform and guide the behaviour and decision-making of people, social groups and those in professions such as nursing. More generally, values are statements about what is seen as good or desirable in a group or specific social or cultural setting.

Values are associated with a particular way or pattern of behaviour that is seen as right or ethical by the individual or others who subscribe to them. Our values are derived from many sources. For example, we develop personal values from parents, siblings and others close to us. In addition, our values are extended and developed through contact with friends, teachers and work colleagues. Although we develop many of our core values during childhood and adolescence, a person's values can change over time due to exposure to new ideas, having new experiences and being influenced by others whom we find charismatic, persuasive and authoritative. Personal reflection is also important in helping us to think through and sometimes revise our values.

Nursing as a profession has had a long-standing interest in values. Nurses are influenced by their own personal values but must also incorporate the collective values of the nursing profession into their practice and behaviour. The Nursing and Midwifery Council code of conduct incorporates and expresses the core values of nursing and is used to guide and regulate the behaviour of registered nurses in practice. The basic aim of the code of conduct is to ensure that nurses apply values that primarily focus on the needs of the people they provide care for. In doing so, the values of nursing practice will promote and protect the interests of those receiving care at a point in their life when they are vulnerable and may be unable to meet their own needs independently.

Social scientists recognise that values make you who you are, motivate your behaviour and guide your personal and professional choices and decision-making. All nurses need to be aware of and understand their own values to appreciate why they do what they do. This is particularly important when a patient's values differ from, or conflict with, those of the nurse. In these situations it is important to find a balance between the patient's rights and the nurse's professional and legal duties (Fry and Johnstone, 2008).

See also – Ethics

Reference and further reading

Baillie, L. and Black, S. (2014) *Professional Values in Nursing*. Boca Raton, FL: CRC Press.

Cuthbert, S. and Quallington, J. (2017) *Values and Ethics for Care Practice*. Banbury: Lantern Publishing.

Fry, S. and Johnstone, M-J. (2008) *Ethics in Nursing Practice: a guide to ethical decision making*, 2nd edition. Oxford: Blackwell.

Violence (and aggression)

Violence is "the intentional use of physical force or power, threatened or actual, against oneself, another person, or against a group or community, which either results in or has a high likelihood of resulting in injury, death, psychological harm, maldevelopment or deprivation" (World Health Organization). Violence is often preventable, particularly where it is triggered by excessive consumption of alcohol.

A number of different factors have been identified as a way of explaining why people sometimes use violent behaviour. These can be divided into innate, socialisation and situational factors.

Table 16 – Factors influencing violent behaviour

Type of factor	Explanation
Innate	• Aggression and violence are seen by biological psychologists as evolutionary instincts 'hard wired' into human beings as survival mechanisms and linked to testosterone levels • Psychoanalytical theory sees aggression and violence as an inborn tendency or drive to destroy; part of the death wish, but also linked to a survival instinct • Neuropsychologists argue that increased aggression and violent behaviour can result from a damaged and dysfunctional brain
Socialisation	• Behavioural psychologists argue that reinforcement of aggressive and violent behaviour by parents and siblings increases the likelihood of violent behaviour later in life • Social learning theory suggests that observation of aggressive and violent behaviour by role models legitimises this kind of behaviour and leads to imitation
Situational	• People living in overcrowded areas with high levels of poverty and fewer opportunities are more likely to experience and use aggression and violence in everyday life • Pain, frustration, loud noises, alcohol and hot environments are also situational factors that may combine with innate and socialised factors to trigger aggressive and violent responses • Normally non-violent people are more likely to behave aggressively and act violently when they are part of a group that behaves in a similar way

See also – Behaviour; Behaviourism

Further reading

Ray, L. (2011) *Violence and Society*. London: SAGE Publications.

Welfare

A dictionary definition of 'welfare' says that it means "well-being; help given to people in need" (*Collins English Dictionary*, 1995). This definition expresses two important, and slightly different, ways of understanding 'welfare' that are also reflected in how people approach social policy.

The first part of the definition says that 'welfare' means 'wellbeing'. In turn 'wellbeing' might be seen to mean things such as the sense of security, happiness and comfort that people seek or want and perhaps even have a 'right' to in their daily lives. A desire to improve the wellbeing of individuals who belong to certain social groups is often given as a reason for the development of healthcare and social policies and can be the focus of healthcare practice.

The second part of the dictionary definition of 'welfare' suggests that it has something to do with the 'help given to people in need'. Sealey (2015) identifies five main areas of basic human welfare needs: health, education, housing, income maintenance and personal social care. A welfare need can be seen as something that is a necessity for life (e.g. food, water, shelter) as well as

something that can enhance the quality of a person's life (e.g. education). Social policies do focus on the creation and delivery of 'welfare *services*' (help) to meet the welfare needs of particular groups of people (those 'in need'). The welfare services typically provided in this way are state-funded health and social services. These may be delivered by statutory organisations or by private or independent sector organisations who have been commissioned to do this on behalf of the state. As such, statutory health and social policies tend to focus on providing services that aim to protect and support those social groups whose members *lack* wellbeing. These include, for example, people who are experiencing poverty and people who have health problems.

See also – Citizenship; Community; Social model of health; Social policy; Welfare state

Reference and further reading

Alcock, P., Haux, T., May, M. and Wright, S. (2016) *The Student's Companion to Social Policy*, 5th edition. Chichester: John Wiley & Sons.

Hills, J. (2015) *Good Times, Bad Times: the welfare myth of them and us*. Bristol: Policy Press.

Sealey, C. (2015) *Social Policy Simplified: connecting theory and concepts with people's lives*. Basingstoke: Palgrave Macmillan.

Welfare state

The National Health Service (NHS) and a national system of social security provision were developed by a Labour government following the recommendations of Sir William Beveridge in the Beveridge Report (1942) on the social problems affecting Britain following the Second World War. This system of state-funded and state-provided healthcare and welfare services is often referred to as the 'welfare state'.

The aim of the 'welfare state' was to tackle the five 'giant evils' of poverty – ill health, lack of education, poor housing and unemployment – that affected the 'welfare' of British citizens in the 1930s and 1940s. Developing the 'welfare state' system in the post-war period involved a massive increase in the amount and scope of state intervention in the provision and funding of welfare. Between the end of the Second World War and the late 1970s, there was a general political consensus that state intervention and funding of welfare was a good thing. During the 1970s, an economic crisis and the emergence of new political ideas that challenged the intervention of the state in people's everyday lives ultimately led to the breakdown of the post-war consensus that viewed the 'welfare state' as a good thing.

The welfare state is based on the idea that there should be equality of opportunity, an equitable distribution of wealth and that the state has a responsibility to ensure that people unable to care for themselves or meet their own needs independently are protected and supported. In practice, the welfare state involved the government providing large amounts of funding acquired through taxation to organisations such as the NHS and local authorities to provide services and social security benefits at a minimum income level to those in need. As part of the welfare state, the NHS was founded on three key principles in 1948:

- Services would be free at the point of delivery
- It would be comprehensive in terms of covering all people in all areas of the country
- Access to services would be on the basis of 'real' – that is clinical – need, rather than the ability to pay, chance or other social criteria.

See also – Community; Social policy; Welfare

Further reading

Fraser, D. (2017) *The Evolution of the British Welfare State*, 5th edition. Basingstoke: Palgrave Macmillan.

Garland, D. (2016) *The Welfare State: a very short introduction*. Oxford: Oxford University Press.